EROTIC

massage

EROTIC
massage

SENSUAL TOUCH FOR DEEP PLEASURE & EXTENDED AROUSAL

Charla Hathaway

QUIVER

Text and photography © 2007 by Quiver

First published in the USA in 2007 by
Quiver, a member of
Quayside Publishing Group
33 Commercial Street
Gloucester, MA 01930
www.quiverbooks.com

11 10 09 08 07   1 2 3 4 5

ISBN-13: 978-1-59233-260-1
ISBN-10: 1-59233-260-9

Library of Congress Cataloging-in-Publication Data
Hathaway, Charla.
  Erotic massage : sensual touch for deep pleasure and extended arousal
/ Charla Hathaway.
      p. cm.
   ISBN-13: 978-1-59233-260-1
   ISBN-10: 1-59233-260-9
  1. Sex instruction. 2. Massage. I. Title.
   HQ31.H38 2007
   613.9'6—dc22

                              2006101421

Cover design by Michael Brock
Book design by Holtz Design
Photography by Allan Penn Photography
Author photo by Wade H. B. Matthews, Jr.

Printed and bound in Singapore

DEDICATION

*For all claiming joy as a touchstone and pleasure
as a path into the wonder of a new world.*

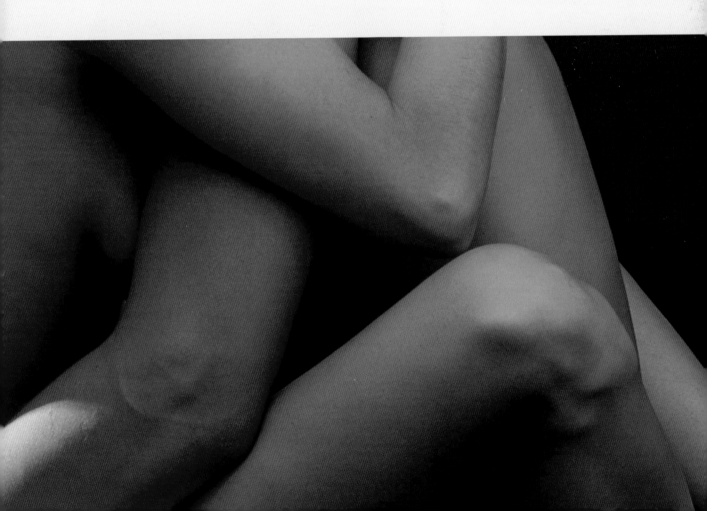

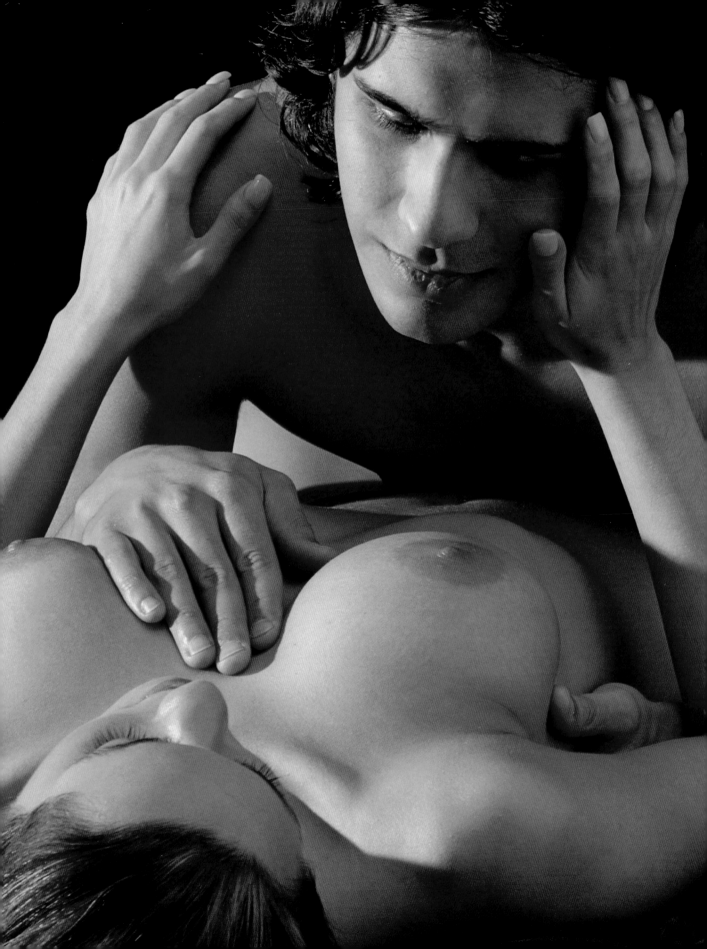

CONTENTS

BODY
time

Welcome to a simple guide into another way of being. I invite you to abandon your thoughts and enter your body senses. Learning to fall effortlessly into the body and spend timeless moments in erotic trance is your birthright. This book is your guide. Each page reclaims forgotten pleasures of your most treasured but least utilized sense—touch. Our bodies are naturally wired for ecstasy. Our sense of touch, unlike the other senses, grows more acute with age, as does our ability to enjoy it. The tools to develop our body's innate ecstasy potential are simple and profound. These techniques are covered in Erotic Massage in a way that's easy to learn and fun to practice!

I will guide you breath by breath, stroke by stroke, into the suspended consciousness of deep surrender for both giving and receiving a sensual massage. Whether you have five minutes or two hours to spare, you'll be inspired to drop into body time every day to relax your mind, energize your body, and elevate your heart.

Warning: This book may be hazardous to your status quo. You can get addicted to body time and need a fix of juicy, in-the-moment touch every day. You may lose your feeling of separateness from your body, as well as your feeling of detachment from your partner. You may claim a new comfort and appreciation for your being, and a desire to share it more often with your lover! Reading this book is your commitment to embracing your ecstatic nature.

I encourage you to pursue more pleasure in life, a message we don't often hear at home, school, work, or church. You can cultivate and embody greater levels of erotic energy in your body than you ever imagined. I know this from personal experience. I was over fifty before I learned the techniques of erotic trance that I'm sharing with you in this book. We're never too young or too old to expand our sensuality. The techniques for erotic massage in these pages will guide you clearly and joyfully into expanded pleasure, healthy well-being, and even personal transformation.

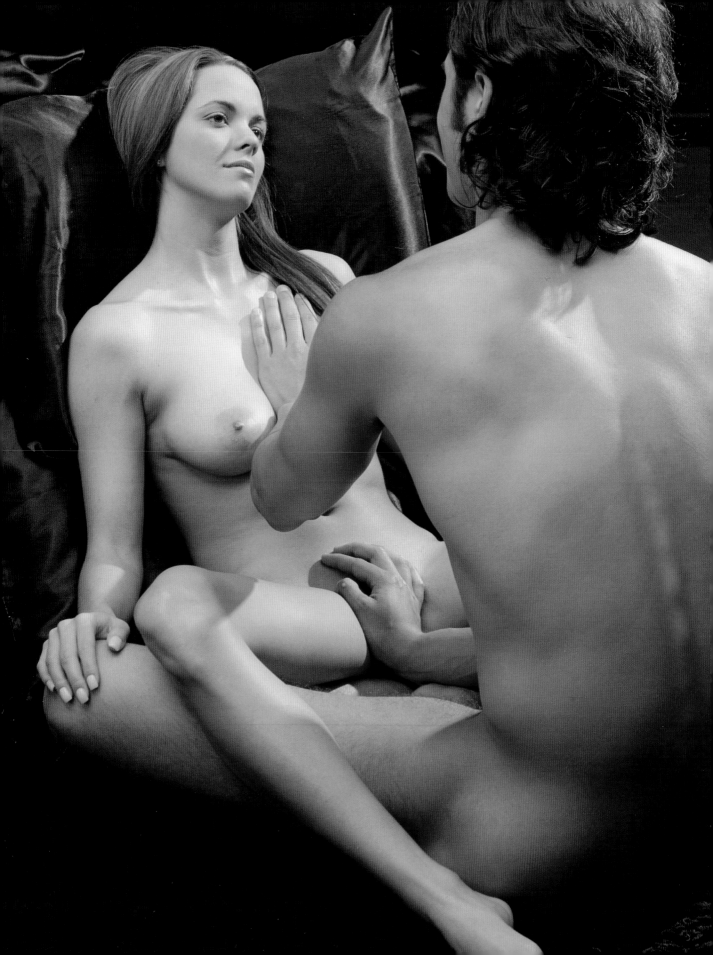

I want to demystify massage and enable you to learn many massage activities that you may choose to share with a partner, or perform by yourself, whenever you're in the mood for sensual touch.

Massage is spiritual food. We start with simple caresses of the hand or face that take only ten minutes out of a busy day. You'll learn to communicate your preferences and express your desires before we move on to full body massages and genital touch.

By committing to time frames and expressing boundaries for each massage, you learn to build trust and compliance with your partner. When we know what to expect in an activity, we can let our guard down and begin to feel. Until we feel *safe*, nothing is erotic! You'll become a child again, discovering and playing with the body erotic. You'll delight in touching for your *own* pleasure and being aware of the wonder of life in each breath. You'll learn how to take turns as the giver or the receiver of touch in each activity to deepen your awareness of each other's bodies.

The adult child in you will remember how to play without strings attached. You'll practice touch without the need to go someplace, touch without payback, touch without pressure to perform, and touch without obligation. You'll learn free touching where the mind is focused only on the sensation in the present moment.

Learning to lusciously touch yourself expands your enjoyment of being touched by a partner. By revolutionizing your self-loving (masturbation) techniques, you can bring a new depth and eroticism to partner genital massage. Self-erotic massage in front of your partner is a hot way to transform old inhibited routines into new freedom and bliss.

If you are ready to relax your mind and come to your senses, follow me breath by breath, stroke by stroke, into the heart of your loving.

If you are tired of *thinking* all the time, massage will guide you into *observing*.

If you are tired of *controlling* all the time, massage will lead you into *surrender*.

If you are tired of *achieving* all the time, massage will lead you into *being*.

If you are ready to luxuriate in the awe and wonder of each juicy moment, let's get started. While this book is designed for couples, most exercises can also be practiced alone. Based on the photo, I'll be addressing either a man or a woman throughout the book, but the massage techniques usually are not gender-specific. My suggestion to you is to first read each chapter and then perform the exercises sequentially until you feel comfortable with them. When rereading the book, feel free to pick and choose randomly.

Most of us long to touch and be touched in a timeless, heartfelt way. We long to feel accepted and cherished for the erotic, sensual beings we are. Erotic massage has been my path to greater freedom and grace. I invite you to journey into the heart of your being.

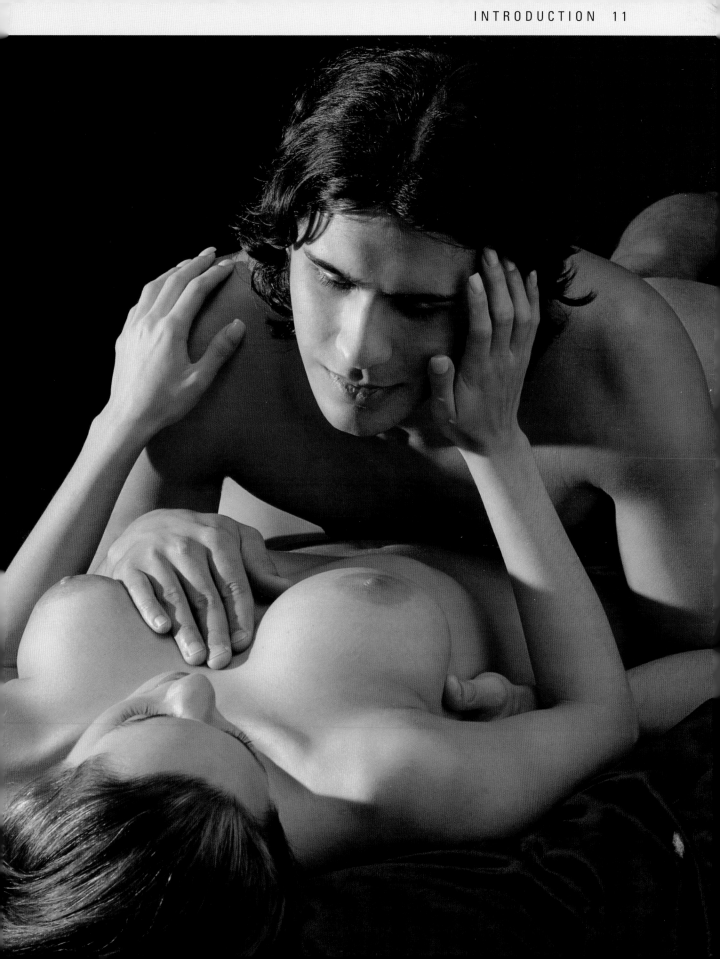

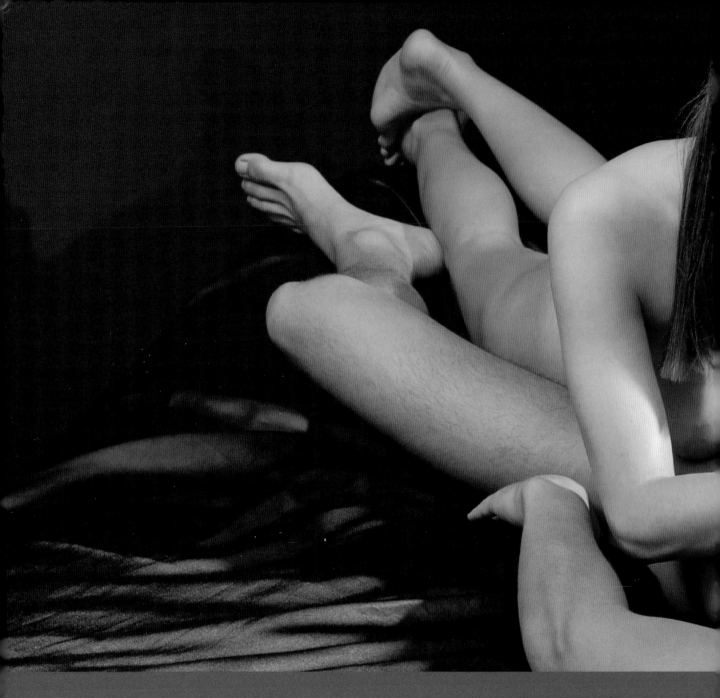

chapter

ONE

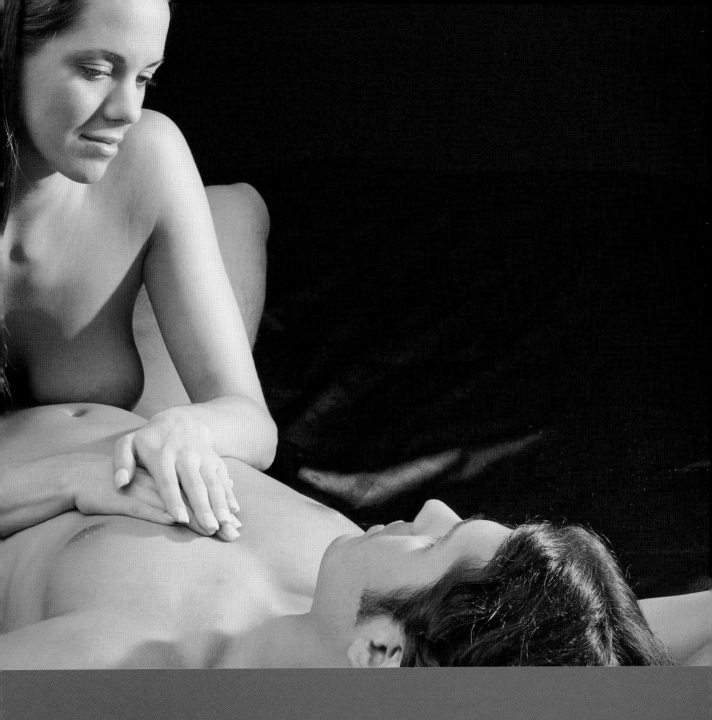

SHOWING UP FOR PLEASURE

Saying yes to pleasure is an acquired skill in our culture. Having fun every day is not usually written into our agenda. Our knee-jerk reaction to pleasure is, "Sounds nice, but I don't have time." Unfortunately, we don't do pleasure well.

How many of us get touched enough in our daily lives? When we were babies, we were held, rocked, and touched all day long. Do we really believe that as adults we don't need it anymore? In our busyness, do we hide a deep hunger to feel cherished, appreciated, and desired?

How can a hardworking, touch-starved person become a rested, touch-fed person? Do we need a doctor's order? "You look frazzled; go home and languish in the arms of your beloved till restored." Do we need a boss's order? "Sales are down; go home, take a long sensual shower, massage yourself, and start daydreaming."

We all remember being "caught" daydreaming as a child and reprimanded by a parent or teacher: "Quit daydreaming; you're wasting time." However, what was being wasted in that time? Maybe being busy all the time is a waste of time. We call ourselves human beings, but we never seem to get around to "being." We're a world full of human doers. And in our frenetic doing and achieving, how much joy and freedom do we feel?

Often our fearful, dualistic thinking leads us to believe we have to choose between two extremes. In this book, I want to show you that you don't have to decide between a life of hard work or pleasure; rather, it's possible to have both! Balance enriches our lives, and it's important to relish in body wisdom and joy everyday.

PERMISSION FOR MORE PLEASURE

As a sex and intimacy coach, my most important job is to give people permission to have more fun. I'm a pleasure activist. My mantras are "Choose fun. Do it for you. Have it your way. Say yes to desires—and express them!" I encourage women to flirt, turn themselves on, and brag. I help men trade in their intellectual minds and preoccupation with "doing" for some enjoyment of the moment and feeling in their bodies. I see a softness wash over the faces of my clients, a liveliness and hope returning, and the hidden girl or boy comimg out to play. I've seen it, and I love watching it happen.

I like to imagine a world serious about pleasure. You greet a friend excitedly: "Want to hear about the greatest orgasm I had last night?" Or, "The funniest thing happened when I was self-pleasuring in the laundry room this morning." Or, teasingly, "Did I ever tell you my fantasy about . . . ?" We're all ears. We're kids at heart. When did we stop playing? When can we start again?

Erotic massage will elevate your pleasure ceiling. If you experience boredom and routine in your life, I prescribe a regular dose of touch—the sensual, no-pressure, no-destination kind of touch. I suggest you schedule some time—five, ten, or twenty minutes most days (and occasionally longer) to explore the body erotic with massage activities in this book. Pleasure is a discipline. Put it on the schedule.

Touching is the gateway into our hearts.

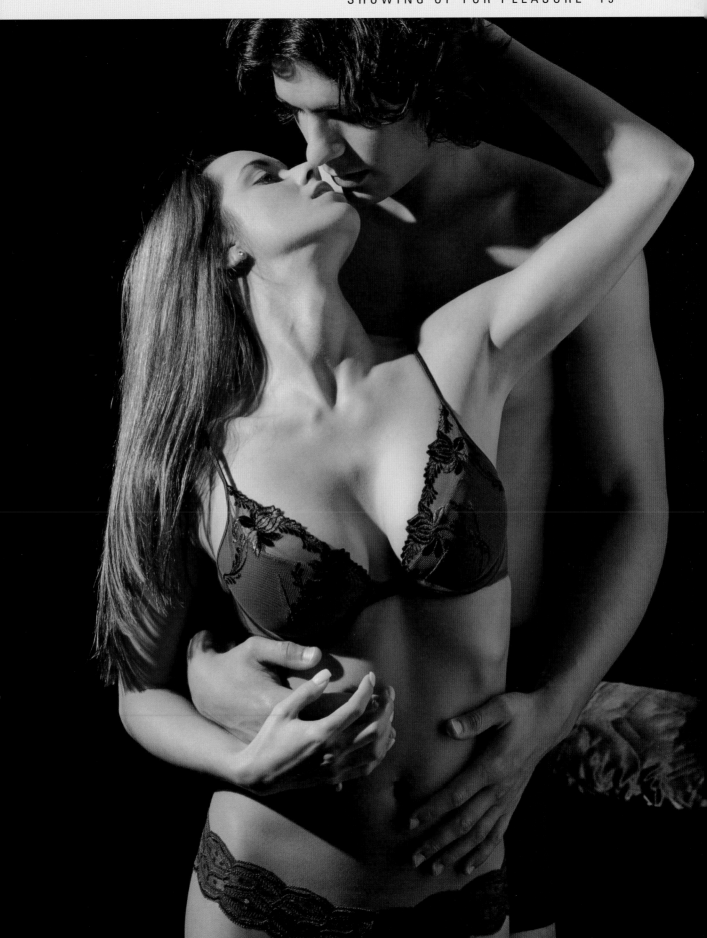

BREATHING AND THE BODY ELECTRIC

Learning simple breathing techniques is the key to enjoying an erotic massage. Conscious breathing teaches you to rid the mind of chatter and the need to "perform" for your partner. Awareness of your breath can move erotic energy generated in one area, such as the genitals, into an electrifying *whole-body* experience.

Conscious breathing slows the mind, deepens touch sensations, and suspends ordinary time. By focusing on the breath, we can experience a deep, nourishing embodiment. Our sense of separateness melts, self-doubt evaporates, and we simultaneously feel energized and relaxed. Focusing on your breath becomes the pathway to connection with your partner and the entire cosmos.

We in the West have overlooked how awareness of the breath, long practiced by the mystics of many traditions, is a simple yet profound tool for personal transformation. You may be surprised how practicing ocean breathing can bring immediate and powerful changes.

OCEAN BREATHING: SOLO

Ocean breathing is a slow, even, deep breathing with an occasional sigh of "Ahhhh" on the exhale. It's a sure pathway into erotic surrender or trance, whether you're giving or receiving an erotic massage.

Practice ocean breathing by constricting your nostrils slightly on the *inhale*, so you can hear the airstream coming in through your nose. Remember when you were a child and someone put a shell up to your ear and said, "Listen, you can hear the ocean inside"? That's the sound you make through your nose with each inhale. Let your relaxed abdomen rise with the inhale, and allow your mind to follow the ocean sound of your breath all the way into your belly.

On the *exhale*, open your mouth slightly and let out an "Ahhhh" as if you were fogging up a mirror with your moist, warm exhale. Soften your throat and feel the vibrations as you sigh or moan on the exhale. Try placing your hand over your throat to feel the vibrations. Let the sound flow out effortlessly through the open throat.

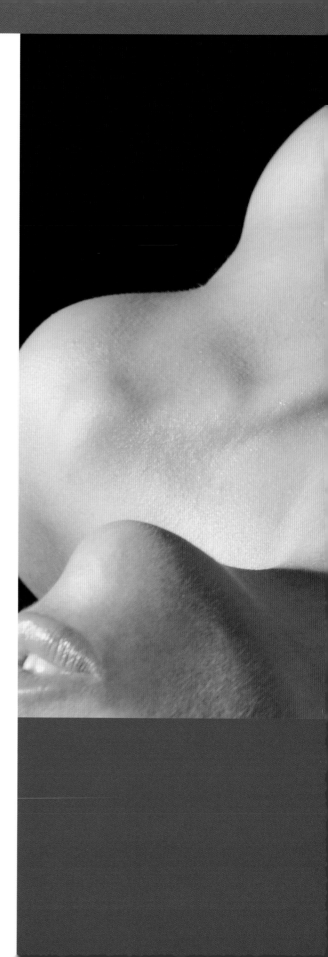

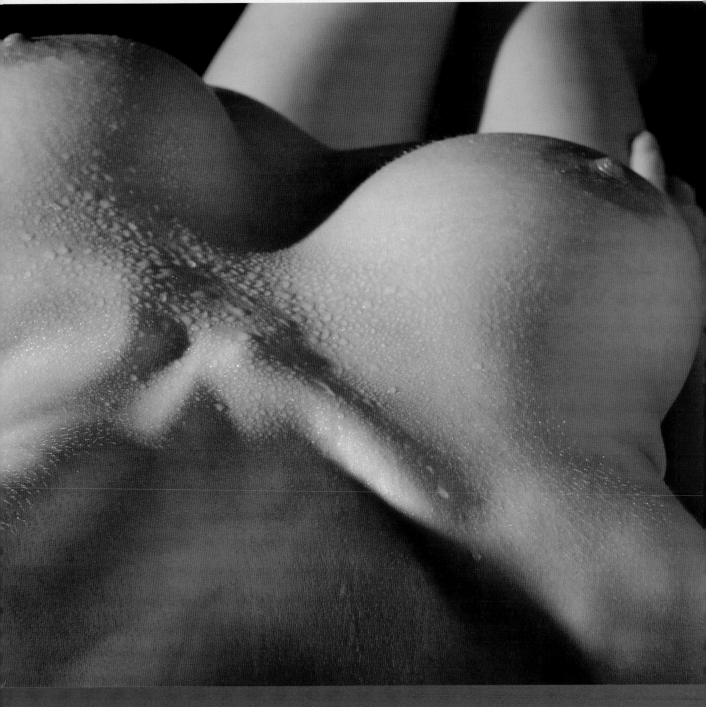

When you and your partner practice conscious
breathing, your sense of separateness melts and
you simultaneously feel energized and relaxed.

Learn to "ride the sound" of each breath by following with your mind the air coming in and falling out of the body. Keep your belly soft. Direct your mind, over and over again, to follow the sound of each breath. Yogis know that if you can hear your breath and can follow it, you are in the present moment. Meditative and spiritual sexuality practices such as Tantra (the yoga of sex) start with awareness of the breath. Ecstatic massage is no different. Breath is your ticket to ecstasy.

Set a timer for five minutes and sit comfortably to practice ocean breathing. Timers keep us from distracting ourselves by watching a clock. This gentle exercise can feel like coming home to yourself—even making gentle love to yourself. Developing a daily practice of ocean breathing strengthens your ability to let go of the mind and recede into your body during a massage.

"You know the feeling you get from orgasm after sex, not the energy rush but the peaceful, melancholy feeling that nothing in the world bothers you? That's what the eye contact, breathing, and focus of my girlfriend's touch during my full body massage did for me. Not only was all the tension in my muscles gone, but I also felt a little purified."
—Tom, 32

OCEAN BREATHING FOR TWO

Set the timer for five minutes. Sit across from your partner cross-legged with your knees touching (with or without clothes on), or with the woman sitting on the man's lap. Look into the left eye of your partner with a soft *gaze*. Be aware of the space behind your eyes. Notice your breathing. Is it slow and deep, or fast and irregular? Gradually synchronize your breathing and hold each other's gentle gaze.

Begin ocean breathing together, listening to both your and your partner's inhale and exhale. If her breath is inaudible, ask her to make more sound. We have been taught to breathe silently, so breathing in a more vocal manner may be an obstacle some people may have to overcome. Find a slow rhythm that is comfortable for both of you. Enjoy the permission to gaze upon your beloved, sharing the same breath, and making sound together. When your mind wanders, gently return your attention to the breath.

Be willing to tap into another way of being. Often our mind resists at some point and wants to regain control. Right beyond this point awaits *trance*—an expansive and delicious state. You can assure the thinking mind that you will return after a few minutes of observing the breath. You soon will look forward to taking a break from ordinary consciousness by ocean breathing. Your power of concentration and attention will need to be exercised. If you're patient, the rewards will be great.

End the ocean-breathing session with a heart salutation. Place your hands together in prayer position at your heart, your thumbs touching the breastbone. Inhale deeply with your partner, then lean forward toward each other, exhaling as the middle of your foreheads touch at the third eye (also called the *mind's eye*, which is our center of intuition). A heart salutation honors the divine spark in each of us and brings closure to the many activities you'll be practicing in this book.

"I'd never really looked at Natalie like that before taking the time to really see her. I guess we usually don't give ourselves that permission to really see one another. Letting our thoughts go and breathing in sync, I felt relaxed and transported."
—Randy, 34

Ocean breathe with your partner by synchronizing your breathing and holding each other's gentle gaze.

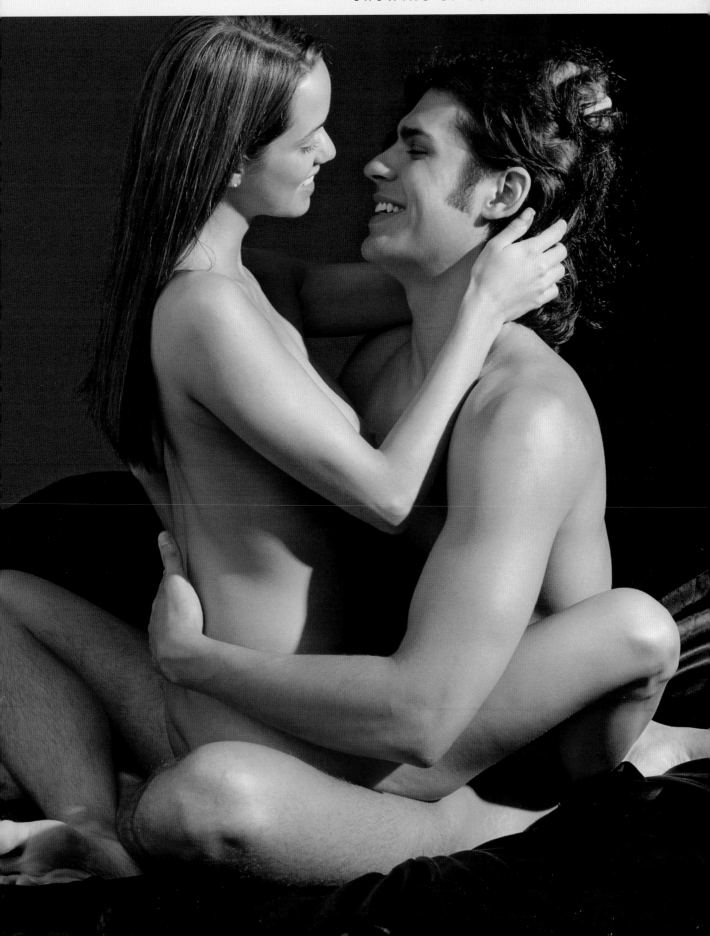

CREATING A **SEXY** SPACE

Years ago I received an original, artistic invitation in the mail from my husband inviting me to a "Night of Sensual Ecstasy." I was returning home after a couple of months away, and he certainly caught my attention. On that special night, he pampered me with a bubble bath, read me poetry, and hand-fed me raspberries laced with cognac. Then he carried me into our bedroom for an erotic massage. To my surprise, I could hardly recognize our room.

Huge pillows adorned the bed, which had been dressed up in new satin sheets. He had redecorated the walls with new photographs of us—some nude—and other erotic artwork (all beautifully framed). Candlelight and soft music gave the room the scent and glow of an ancient temple. A splay of peacock feathers, rabbit fur, exotic misters, lotions, and oils graced the nightstand. Astounded, I gazed through watery eyes at the sacred temple he had created for us.

Our transformed bedroom signaled the internal transformation in our lives. We were committing to more pleasure. Our new sexy bedroom was a metaphor for our new sexy attitude about raising the pleasure ceiling in our marriage. When I would pass through the room in the daytime, I'd stop, reflect, and smile. The space held our passion.

Create your own sexy space in your home for your erotic encounters, whether or not you have a partner. Activity follows intention. Make your space unique— let it be an erotic testament to your desires, history, stories, tastes, and passions. Decorate it all at once or spread the effort out over time, but make the space reflect your intimate personality. Your sacred temple will provide a juicy place for exploration into erotic massage. Just passing by the door will make you smile.

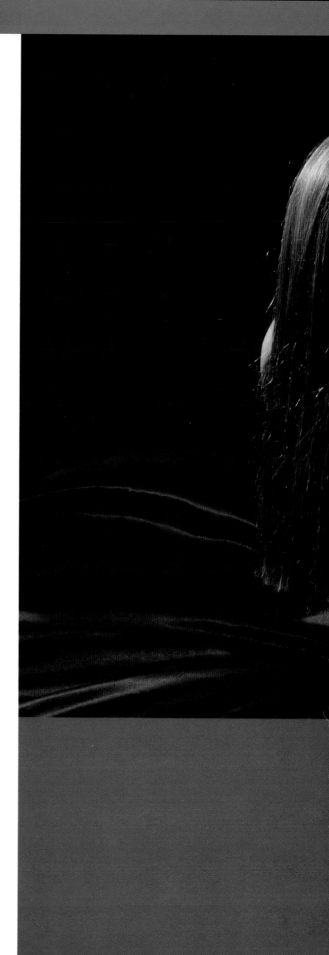

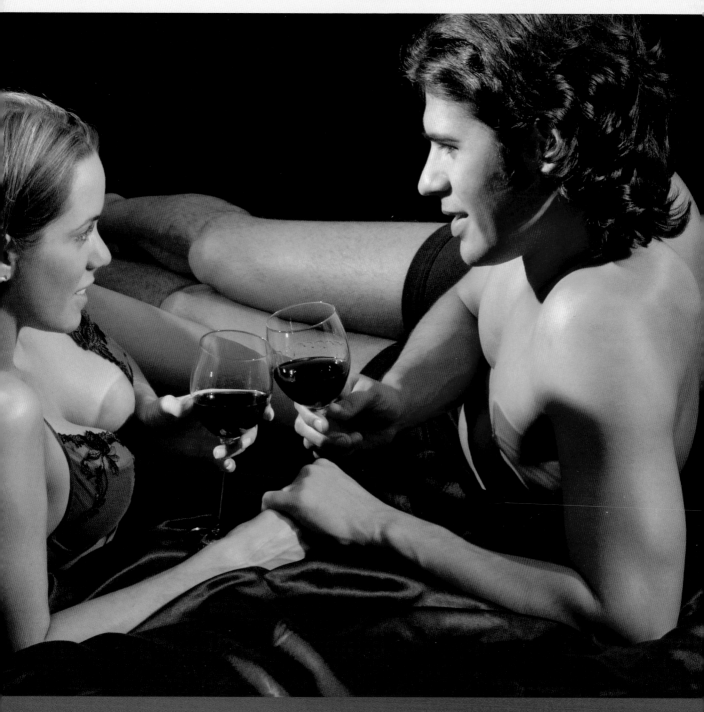

Part of enjoying your lover is taking the time to relax, create, and enjoy your sexy space.

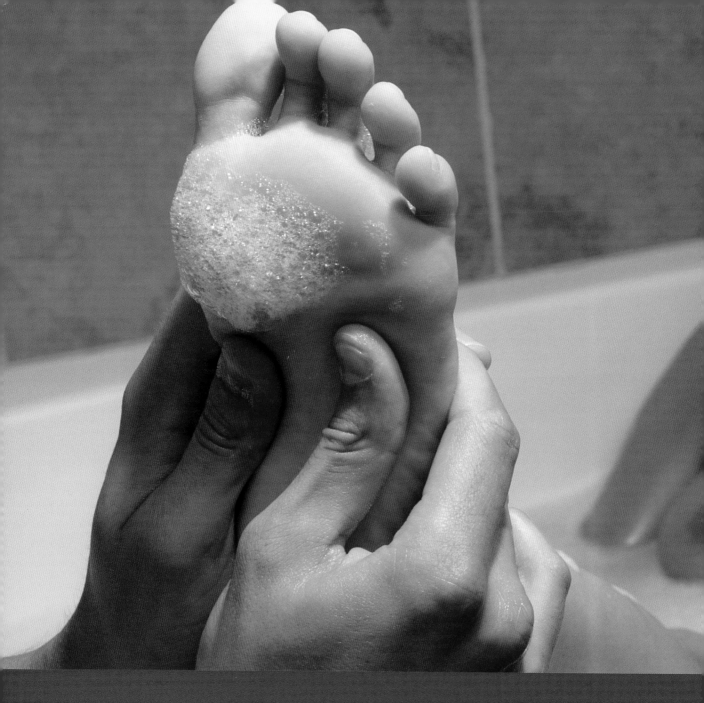

chapter
TWO

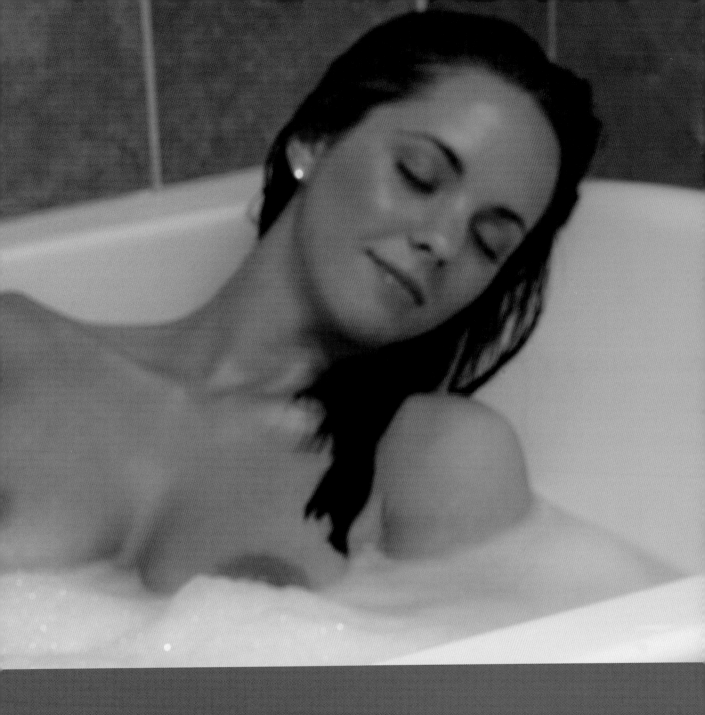

BODY CARESSES

The skin is the largest organ of the body, and as we mature, it grows more sensitive to touch. We can actually feel more than when we were younger, because we're willing to slow down and take time to notice nuances of sensation. Deep awareness of touch relaxes us into erotic trance. Caresses to the hands and the feet send stimuli directly to the sexual organs. Touching these areas produces a subtle buildup of erotic energy.

Body caresses are more sensual than sexual. Sensual touch is about enjoying the pleasure of the sensations in the moment, where sexual touch is more goal-oriented. Although sexual touch can be a natural outcome of sensual touch, in this book we are learning sensual touch, or touch for pleasure in the moment, versus touch that has a destination, such as sexual intercourse. Instead of wanting to reach the goal of sex, you will become enthralled with the journey.

TAKING TURNS

For the exercises in this book, you will first choose to be either the active or the passive partner, then will later switch roles. Taking turns allows you to slow down and really take note of what is happening. When you are the active partner, or the *giver of touch*, you can focus fully on the sensations that your fingertips or hands receive from touching your partner's skin. When you're the passive partner, or the *receiver of touch*, you can be totally aware of each subtle sensation of touch you take in. Alternating being active and being passive allows maximum pleasure, because you'll have time to observe sensations in a fresh and unhurried manner.

TOUCH FOR YOUR *OWN* PLEASURE

We have learned to touch for someone else's pleasure. In relationships, we're programmed to take care of the other person. Touching for your own enjoyment will seem different, and this new orientation will cultivate vitality, as well as interest, in your caresses. When you are trying to please your partner, you are in performance mode and are therefore anxious about the job you are doing for her. When you're worried about "doing it right," you're not in the present moment. When you touch your partner for your *own* gratification, you will allow yourself to relax and enjoy and thereby invite your partner to do the same.

Accepting Pleasure

Often when we receive touch, we think, "Now that I've taken my share, I have to give back." We feel self-conscious, or selfish, by receiving so much attention. Deep down, maybe we don't think we deserve all that goodness. Taking turns can help us learn to open up to more pleasure, to take more in. Ultimately, we realize, by feeling pleasure in our partner's touch, that we are giving him a precious gift by receiving fully.

Think how much fun it is to pet a dog or a cat. Does it feel guilty for getting so much attention and cut us off? Does it get up in the middle of a petting because it's his turn to give back? We love those critters because they know how to take it in, milk us for all we're willing to give—shamelessly, unabashedly—and that keeps us happy as givers. Give up putting a time limit on your receiving pleasure. Be ardent—even gluttonous—when you are receiving (or giving, for that matter).

Taking turns giving and receiving touch develops focus and presence.

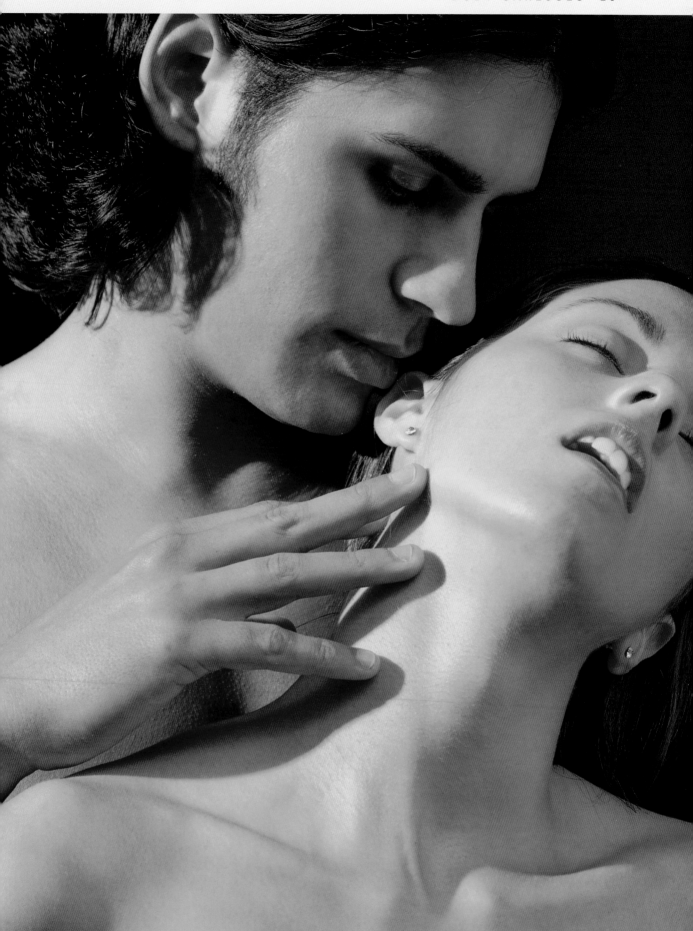

PREPARING FOR A
CARESS

The hands are a great place to start caressing, because they are sensitive, used to being touched, and extend from our heart center, which expresses love. Decide who will give the caress first. Make yourselves comfortable, with or without clothes on, and support your back if desired. Decide on a time frame for the duration of the caress, such as ten minutes, then start the timer.

Do an abbreviated heart salutation in which you bow to each other with your hands at your heart (foreheads need not come together). This gives a formal beginning to the caress. Begin ocean breathing for one or two minutes, gazing softly into the other's left eye (the window of the soul) and following the sound of the breath.

FOCUS ON YOUR SENSATIONS

When the giver is ready, place your partner's hand in yours as you would a precious jewel. Feel the heat between your hands. Feel the weight of the hand. Very slowly begin to trace the outline of the palm and fingers. Close your eyes to better explore each contour, crevasse, line, and fold. Marvel over this hand that has brought you so much pleasure. Fill yourself with awe over the sensory discovery at your fingertips.

Caresses are nonverbal, which encourages your right brain to lead (it functions in a nonverbal manner and excels in visual, spatial, perceptual, and intuitive information). Resist breaking out of this space with the tendency to talk or respond to each other through gestures.

A caress is not a massage. While you are awakening the nerves in the skin, you are not manipulating the muscle tissue underneath. Often the lighter the touch, the more stimulating. Too much pressure and repeated stroking in one area deadens the sensations. Barely touch the hair. The roots go deep, and he'll feel everything.

If you find it hard to stay focused, try touching *more slowly and more lightly*. If you lose your concentration, stop touching, find your breath again, or—even better—breathe with your partner for a couple of breaths. Stillness is as powerful as a stroke. If you catch your partner holding the breath in, breathe gently in his ear to remind him to ocean breathe. The breath slows your mind and helps you stay focused in the present moment, whether you're giving or receiving. Conscious breathing is your anchor.

COMPASSIONATE COMMUNICATION

When you think about half of the time frame has passed, you may want to caress the other hand. The timer will signal the end of this caress. Gently lay the hand down, open your eyes, and complete the caress with a heart salutation. Appreciate how you have honored the hands, the vehicle of our creativity and work in the world. Reset the timer for ten minutes, and change roles.

Take a moment to appreciate your lover's hand and the pleasure that it has brought you.

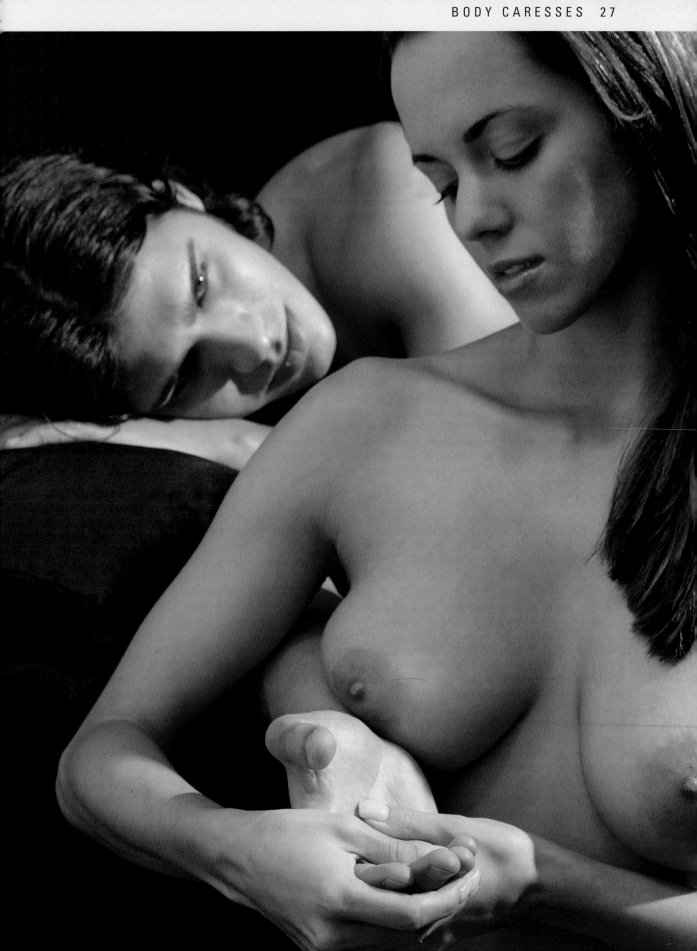

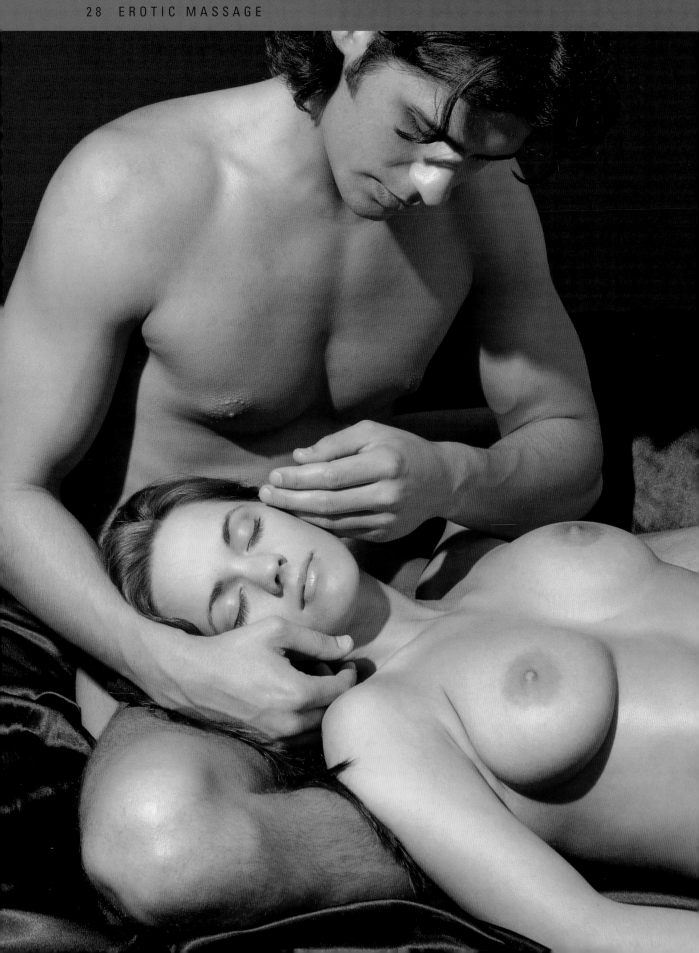

FACE CARESS

Giving your partner a face caress is like seeing her for the first time. Permission to explore the face is an intimate and magical gesture. Decide on who will be active first (the man in this example). Sit comfortably, with your back supported, and lay your partner's head on a pillow in your lap. Set the timer for ten minutes. Gaze softly at each other, and ocean breathe together for a minute or two.

When you are ready, place both of your hands lightly over her entire face. Feel the heat: Be aware of your intent to create wonder with your exploration. With your eyes open (hers may be closed), begin touching her forehead at the hairline. Move your fingers slowly through her hair. Notice the hair slipping between your fingers and underneath your nails. Move to the forehead. Is the skin tight, cool, soft, or warm? Explore each line in the skin with awe, imagining the wisdom from the experience it holds.

Move your fingers over her eyebrows from the center outward. Leisurely retrace your stroke. Touch the very ends of the eyelashes with a fingertip. Encourage your partner to stay deep in the breath by modeling for her *your* slow, even breathing. Touch for your pleasure.

Trace the shape of her cheekbone with your thumb and index finger. Slide down the side of her nose. *Touch with interest.* If your mind wanders from the touch, slow down. An easy mistake is to go too fast. Consider what you experience riding in a car racing down the interstate at 75 mph versus taking a leisurely drive down a country road at 25 mph. Outline the shape of the ear, but don't probe inside. For women, notice the feel of the soft upper cheek versus his whisker stubble or beard. Come to the lips and outline them lightly. The lips may naturally part when touched. Explore this sensual terrain teasingly without probing a finger inside.

Conclude the caress with both hands over the face, then release them slowly. Share a heart salutation and know that the wonder you created in this caress comes from you. Before you switch giver and receiver roles, the receiver should take a moment to share what that experience was like. Use words that can instruct your lover about his touch, such as how his pressure or speed was for you. Discuss what parts you liked best, where he could have lingered longer, and what parts he may have missed.

Touch for your own pleasure,
and do only what pleases you.

Try doing a face caress on yourself. Set aside time, light a candle, and sit in front of a mirror. You are now both giver and receiver. Gaze and breathe—even give yourself a heart salutation. Honor yourself with your own heartfelt touch. Notice how your skin drinks in the sensations. Observe how present you can be with yourself. Close your eyes, lie down if you'd like, and allow the flow of love to come into your being through your fingertips. Give yourself the full time allotted for the caress. You can enjoy all the body caresses as an expression of self-love.

SETTING THE MOOD WITH **INTENTION**

By now you are getting familiar with the opening sequence for starting a caress. You choose either the active or the passive role, decide on a time frame, set the timer, then bow in a heart salutation and connect through ocean breathing. This opening ritual, taking only a few minutes, signals a clear departure from the ordinary day and ordinary time, and the beginning of body time. By repeating the simple ritual, the mind slips more readily into surrender, and the body steps forward to take the lead.

A meaningful addition to this calming sequence is to *set an intention* for your caress. By deciding on an intention, you shape or define your experience more precisely. You'll find that having an intention deepens the experience and can bring you back to noticing body sensations when your mind wanders off. You may intend simply "to listen for each breath," or "to feel a flow of appreciation between you and your partner," or "to feel each sensation," or "to love yourself more deeply." It becomes an anchor that can help return you to the present moment when you get distracted.

We change *ordinary* touch into *sacred* touch simply by our intention to do so. Stating an intention can be done silently to yourself or stated out loud to your partner, which is a more powerful gesture. Be sure to state your intention with *positive language*. For example, if you intend not to worry about the children while getting caressed, say, "I intend to breathe in peace with every inhale."

FOOT CARESS

Our feet are full of nerve endings that connect directly to our sexual organs, making feet highly sensual and erotic organs. The humble gesture of bathing and caressing the feet, in or out of the bathtub, is a most delightful and enjoyable act.

Begin by filling a small tub or pan with warm water and adding some bath salts. Place two towels, soap, and lotion or oil nearby. Once you begin your caress, you will not want to be interrupted by trying to find these items. Place large pillows on the floor for the receiver's comfort, as well as extra pillows for under the knees to support the entire leg.

Choose the active partner (the massage giver), set your timer for twenty minutes, and bow in an honoring heart salutation. Both partners should try to construct a positive, one-sentence intention and express it either silently to themselves or verbally to each other. Gaze and ocean breathe together; enjoy how the familiar ritual grounds you in the body. When ready, the man, in this case, lifts the woman's feet slowly into the tub or pan of water.

Lather her feet with soap and explore the tactile sensations by playing with the feet under water. Take one foot out of the basin and place it on a towel lain over your thigh. Again soap the foot using both hands. Slide a finger between the toes. Feel where they meet the ball of the foot. Tug gently on the toes, letting them slip out between your fingers. Enjoy the slippery skin for your pleasure. Return the foot to the bath, and repeat on the other foot. Move slowly in long, continuous strokes. Coach your partner to breathe fully if her breath is shallow, uneven, or quiet. Intimacy is increased by deep breathing together.

Place the second foot back in the tub and rinse. Take the first foot out and wrap it carefully in a towel like a baby's bunting. Do the same with the second foot. Move the water tub aside to give you a free, unencumbered space for caressing. Dry the first foot unhurriedly, paying special attention to the space between the toes.

Rest the foot on your thigh. Explore the foot with light touching as you did in the hand caresses. If your partner is ticklish, stroke using more pressure and let up when she relaxes. Rub massage oil or lotion on your hands, gently covering the entire foot. Lightly stroke with two hands the top and bottom of the foot simultaneously.

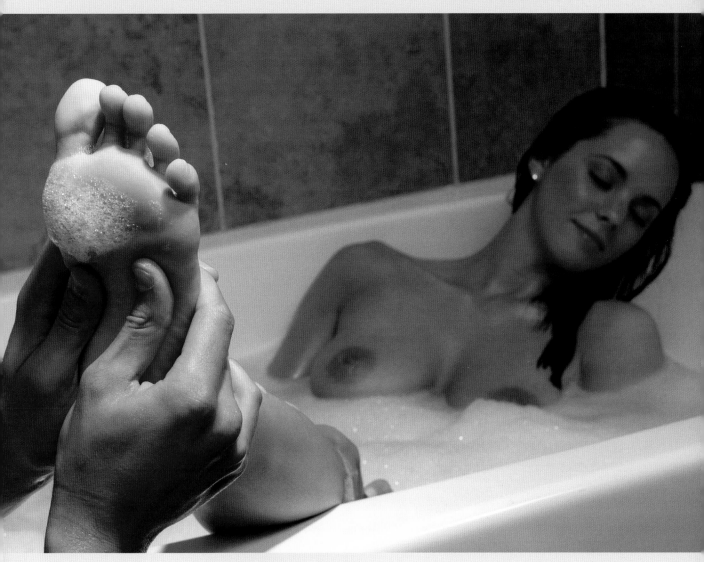

TICKLISHNESS *is often a blockage of sensual*
or sexual energy. If we are ticklish, we cannot be
touched; hence, we are safe from feeling sensations
or becoming sexual. Our feet are particularly
vulnerable, because they are rarely touched but very
sensitive. Remind a ticklish partner to focus on the
point of skin-to-skin contact with a deep breath. Be
patient, and move even more slowly, with a slightly
firmer touch. Return to a lighter touch when possible.
Helping a partner get over blocks to pleasure is
worth the effort.

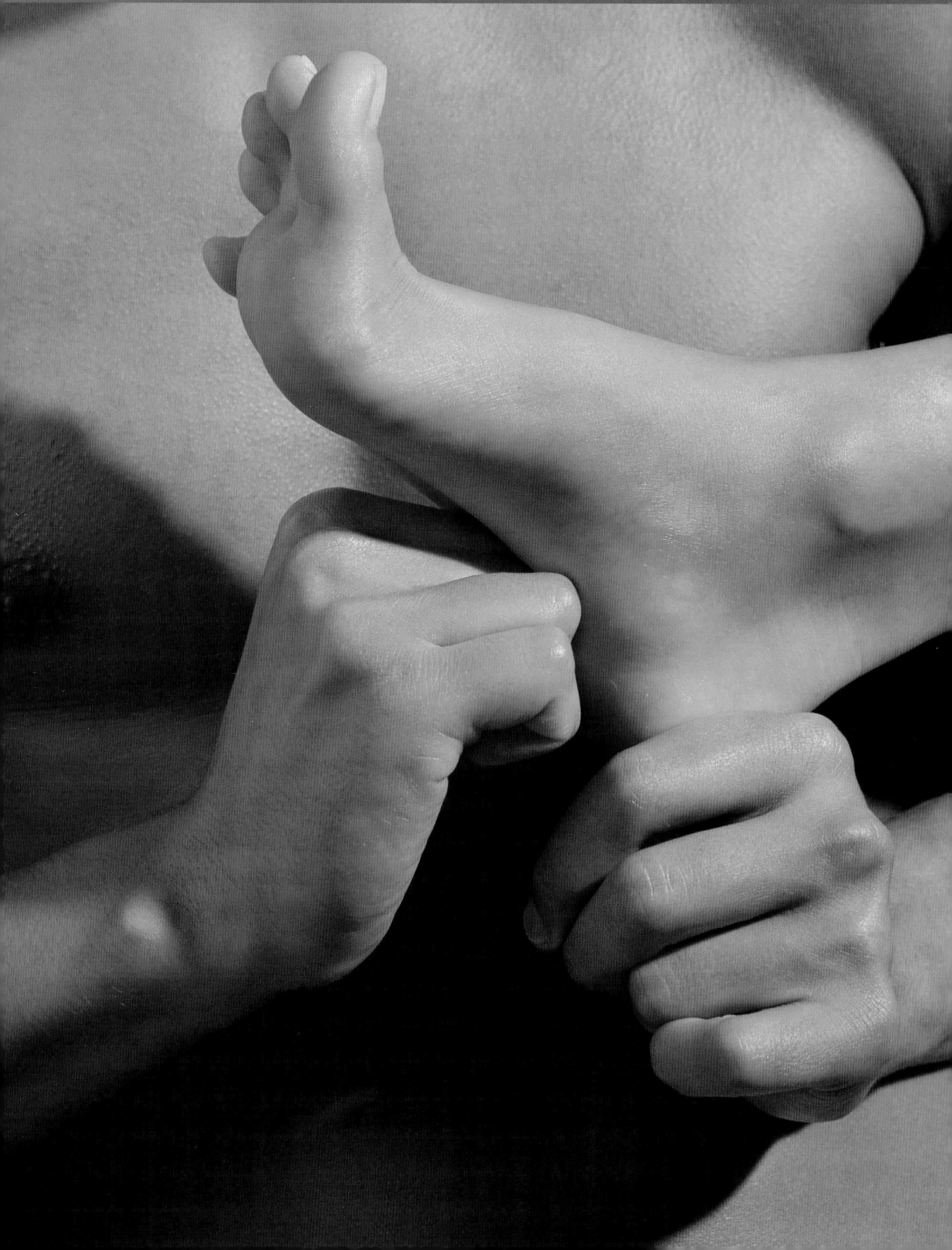

MASSAGE STROKES FOR THE FEET

Massage strokes go deeper than caressing and involve manipulating the underlying muscle tissue. The feet are a perfect starting point. Cap the heel firmly with your hand and massage the ball of the foot with your other hand. Hold the ball of the foot and squeeze the heel till it gradually "pops" out of your grip. Do it several times. Make a fist with the hand at the ball of the foot and firmly glide your knuckles down the center of the bottom of the foot to the heel. Repeat several times. You are activating internal energy channels, or meridians, that send joyous messages to a multitude of organs in the body.

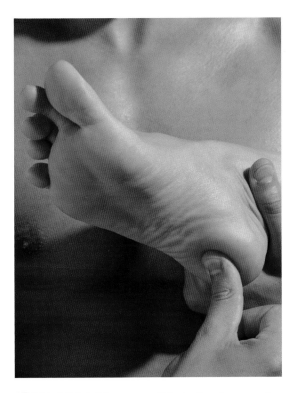

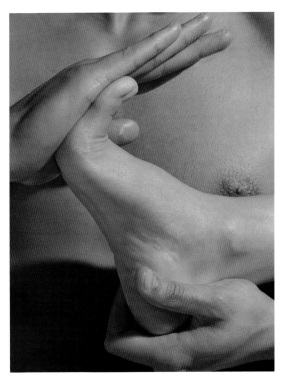

Start at the heel, where you will be indirectly massaging the sexual organs. Use intense pressure (more than you might think), then check in with your partner asking, "Would you like more or less pressure?" Adjust if needed. Continue to play with pressure points on the ball of the foot and between the toes. Tug on each toe, wiggling and pulling on it.

Yoga students use oppositional stretching to rejuvenate the body. Place one palm over the toes, and with the other hold the heel. Press the toes back toward the arch while pulling the heel in the opposite direction. Hold a few moments. Repeat this stretch, pressing deeper, spreading the toes apart with and away from the ball of the foot with your flat palm. With about seven minutes remaining in the massage, change to the second foot.

KISSING THE FEET

Kissing the feet is a gesture of supreme gratitude and servitude; it will melt both you and your partner to the very core. Use your creativity in this area and start delicately. Take the toe(s) inside your mouth and let out a long sigh of hot air without even touching the toes— just a hot-air caress. Stop and feel the heat. Next, flick your wet tongue lightly and playfully over the toe. Pause and take in the moment. Blow a cool stream of air over your hot tongue tracks. Wait. Stillness can be substituted for a stroke. Ask any musician: If they don't play the "rests," there is no music. Go in slightly deeper now. Brush your lips over the surface; slip your tongue in and out between the toes.

Let *your pleasure* guide your licking, nibbling, and sucking. Do not try to impress or perform for her. How does this organ feel on *your* wet, fleshy tongue? What shapes and textures delight *your* sensations? Close your eyes. How does it feel filling your mouth with a part of her? Follow your desire to rhythmically suck and moan and lap up your pleasure. Play like a child—shameless, full of innocence and curiosity.

At the end of the foot massage, gaze into your lover's eyes and notice how erotic energy softens the face. Bow from the heart in gratitude for the timeless and treasured moments you shared. Switch roles and refill the tub with fresh water.

"Sitting across from me at the wedding-rehearsal dinner, a new acquaintance reached for my foot under the table. He slipped off my shoe and began massaging my foot on his knee. While the others thought I was swooning over the silky taste of sushi, we laughed with our friends but kept our secret. When we walked down the aisle the next day, as bridesmaid and groomsman, I was still smiling. To this day, I still cherish this man's simple gift."

—Jennifer, 29

Verbal Massage

The next time you receive a caress, instead of the usual nonverbal exchange, try talking with your partner about how he can make the experience better as he massages you. Tell him more pressure, less pressure, slower, deeper, lighter, over here, or not there, change strokes, etc. After the receiver tells you what he wants or how to do something, respond with, "Thank you." Resist apologizing or defending yourself. Our partner's feedback is a precious gift; a simple "Thank you" acknowledges it as such. None of us are mind readers; we need information to improve our touch techniques.

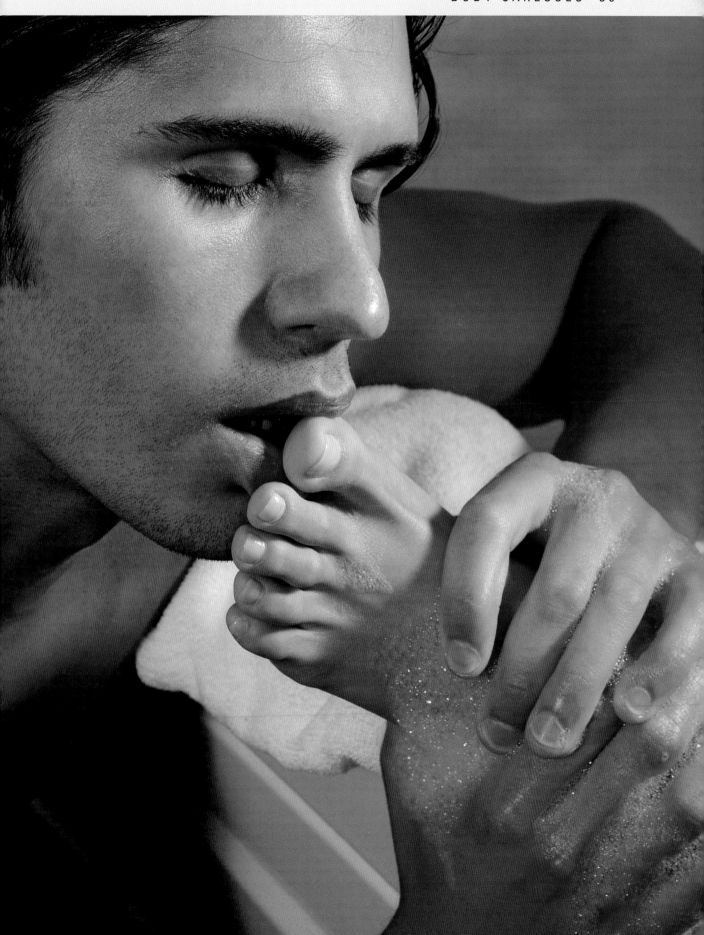

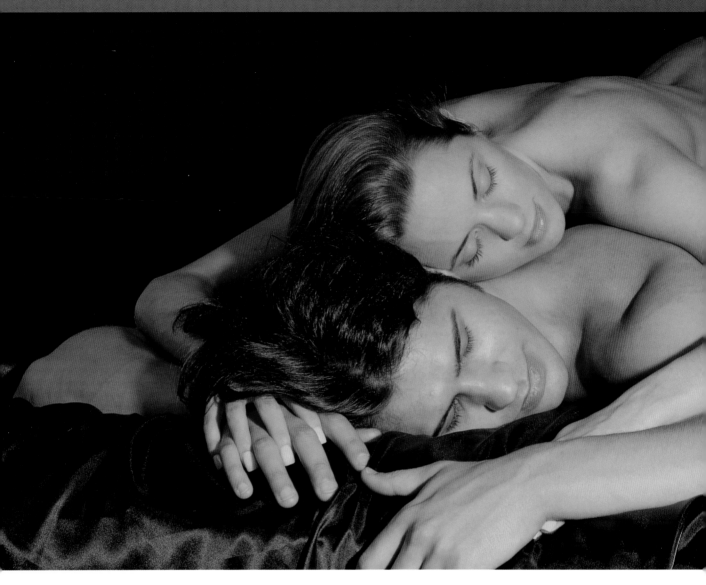

BONDING

Bonding, reminiscent of the warm connection between mother and baby, infuses the entire body with erotic ripples that need not be acted upon in a genital fashion. What looks like inactivity on the surface is perhaps the most profound of all erotic-massage moves. Bonding opens our energy channels at a subtle level where the boundaries between bodies begin to dissolve and merge. Bonding gives us a chance to build and disperse sexual energy with the whole body—not with just the genitals.

Find a comfortable place to lie down together, such as a bed, and set the timer for twenty (or more) minutes. Play some soft, relaxing music. You may lie side by side in a "spooning" position (chest to partner's back), or the lighter partner can lie on top of the heavier one. Make sure you are comfortable and supported by pillows where needed.

Once lying together, begin to be aware of your breath, letting your worries and tension fall away with each exhale. While breathing out, imagine that you are expelling your fears, resentments, and expectations. As you exhale, release the need to think and analyze. Let your tongue float freely in your mouth, not touching any part of the oral cavity. As you inhale, imagine you are filling up with all you need to radiate joy.

Observe your partner's breathing rhythm. It feels

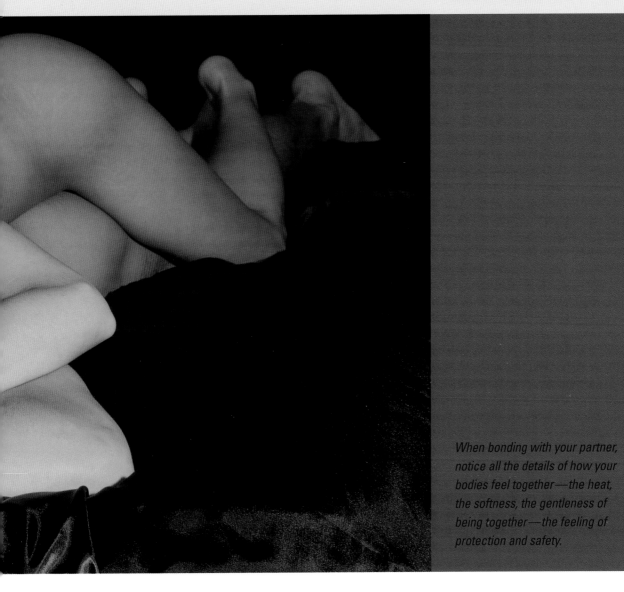

When bonding with your partner, notice all the details of how your bodies feel together—the heat, the softness, the gentleness of being together—the feeling of protection and safety.

natural to breathe together in this ritual. Notice all the details of how your bodies feel together—the heat, the softness, the gentleness of being together, the feeling of protection and safety. With each breath, let yourself fall deeper into the body, becoming transparent; feel the vulnerability of the present moment and the wonder of uncertainty. Feel the new reality where doing and not doing are one, where you allow yourself to melt into the other.

Can you feel your boundaries dissolve into the other? Can your heart open and welcome the other in? Let the exploration be effortless. Can your spirits float away beyond the boundaries of the body? Usually it takes fifteen to twenty minutes (or longer) to deepen

into this formless, relaxed, and merged space. Be patient; even ecstasy needs to be practiced, so repeating this exercise is helpful.

A common mistake is to expect too much too soon. Enjoy the journey. Make sure you feel free to gently readjust your position during bonding. Contrary to your partner's being "disturbed," she will be glad you are making yourself comfortable. End with a heart salutation and mutual sharing of the experience. Relaxation bonding is a stepping-stone to sexual bonding in chapter 8.

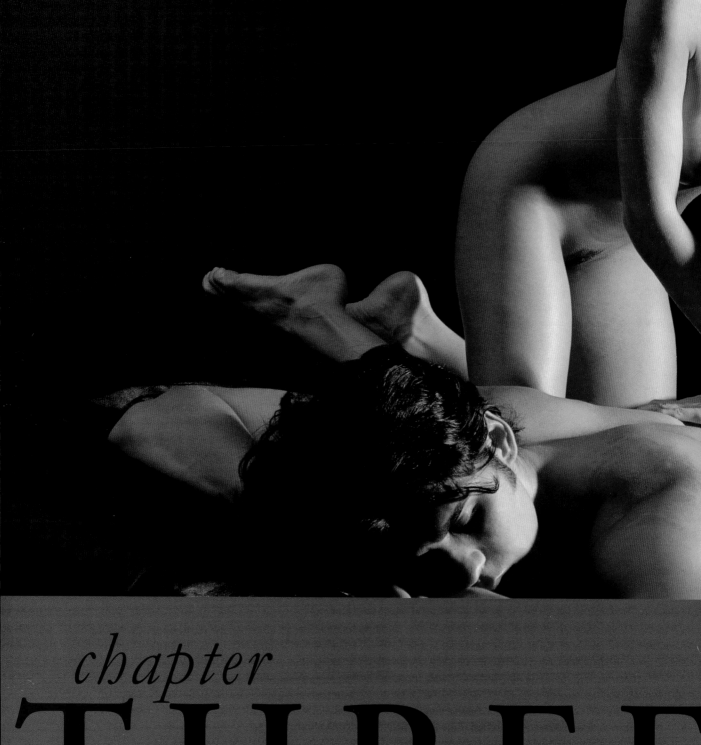

chapter
THREE

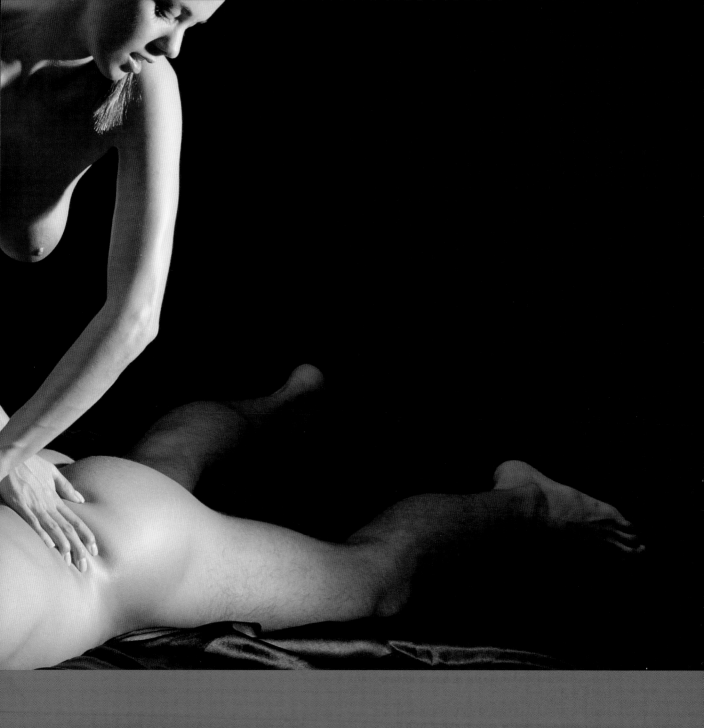

BACK BODY MASSAGE

Body caressing and relaxation bonding practiced in chapter 2 encourage us to linger and luxuriate in the touch. We've begun to feel the energizing and relaxing effects of conscious breathing, touching, and setting intention. These are the keys to cultivating erotic trance, quieting the mind, and opening the heart. In learning back body massage, we will take these erotic tools to a higher level.

In massage we're often concerned about how to give one, how to perform the different strokes, and what to "do" to our partner. Rarely do we concern ourselves with the most challenging part of massage—how to *receive* one. Given our busy culture, we are often more comfortable with doing than with being passive, which can make us feel out of control. The back of the body is the perfect place to practice deeper surrender. We feel safe lying on our stomachs, protecting our vulnerable underbelly, and our genitals are hidden. Feeling safe is necessary before we allow ourselves to surrender.

Couples who have a passionate and satisfying erotic relationship regularly engage in massage as a way to learn surrender. They use sensual massage as a way into sexual play, but, equally satisfying and nourishing, they use erotic massage as a complete activity in its own right. Couples who practice whole-body touching in a playful spirit, whether in the giving or the receiving role, become deeply aware of the ecstasy of surrender. A good intention for this massage may be, "I intend to let each exhale take me deeper into the sensation."

COMING INTO THE BODY

Choose a comfortable bed or soft floor mat in your sexy space and cover it with a protective sheet. Select a quality massage oil or lotion (which can be purchased at any health food store). Play soothing music (without words to distract) and make the ambience inviting with candles and scents.

Set the timer for twenty to thirty minutes. If the man is giving, lie side by side, spooning with the woman in front and his hands over her heart. If the woman is giving (as illustrated in this case), lie on top of the man with your chest on his back. Share a simple, one-sentence intention. Bond and relax by tuning in to your breaths as they rise and fall together. *Enjoy this simplest of rituals—sharing the breath.* Feel a letting go with each exhale, and with each inhale take in a new sense of wonder.

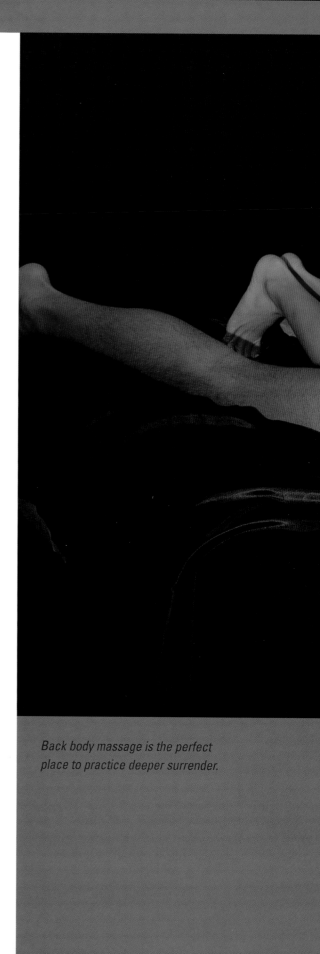

Back body massage is the perfect place to practice deeper surrender.

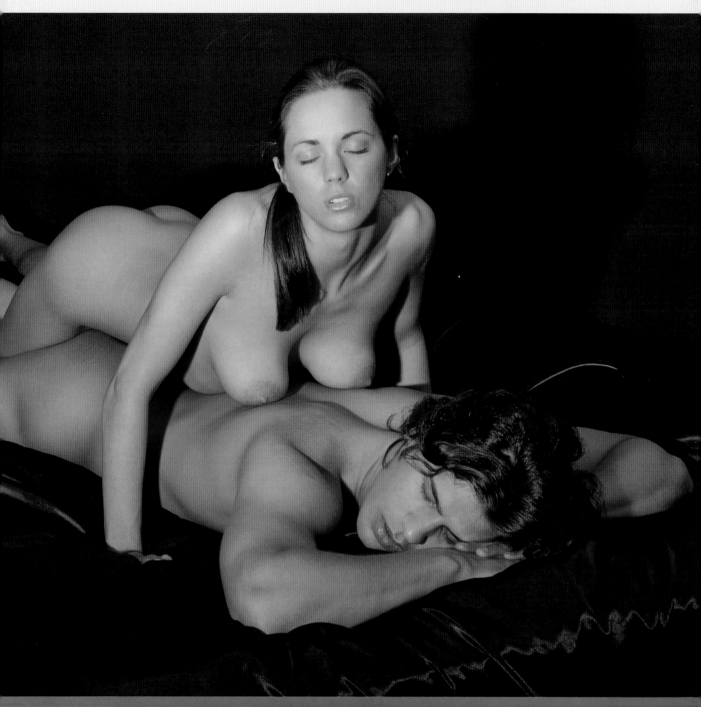

"*At first as a man it was hard for me to just receive. I felt like I needed to initiate or at least give back at the same time. But I stayed with the exercise and soon I relaxed deeply into a new place inside my body. I was grateful for my partner—she genuinely wanted to take care of and give to me.*"

—*Richard, 38*

You can take the breath one step further toward surrender: Make an audible "Ahhhh" sigh on the exhale together. Marvel at how much fun it is to mix your sounds and vibrations. You can lose yourself. You may even laugh together in this position.

After a couple of minutes of grounding and breathing in sync, the woman slowly begins to move her breasts down his back. Let your nipples trace playful designs on his back. Drag your breasts over his buttocks, breathing hot air onto his cool skin. Eventually, kneel between his spread legs.

From this position, reach behind you and place a hand on the bottom of each foot. Using a light touch, with a hand on each leg, simultaneously trace the contour of the calves, stroke up the inner thighs, moving over the buttocks, up each side of the back, over the shoulders, and down the arms to the hands. Use one long, continuous stroke from foot to hand, then reverse it. Repeat a couple of times. See how slowly you can make this awakening stroke.

HEART AND SACRUM HOLD

Kneeling at the man's side, place one hand over his heart and the other hand on his sacrum (the last bone of the spine). These two energetic centers, heart-love and sacrum-sexuality, are energetically connected by simultaneously touching them. Rest your hands on them in stillness and ocean breathe. Listen for his breath. Watch to see the back of his body rise and fall with the breath. If he's holding his breath or shallow breathing, bend over and breathe deeply on his neck. Only when you know where your lover is in the breath are you intimate enough to continue.

Begin a gentle rocking of the body from these two points by moving your hands back and forth about an inch. Be subtle and unhurried, and gradually increase the intensity. The sense of being cherished from this gentle movement is deeply comforting.

A heart-and-sacrum hold will connect your partner's heart and sex centers.

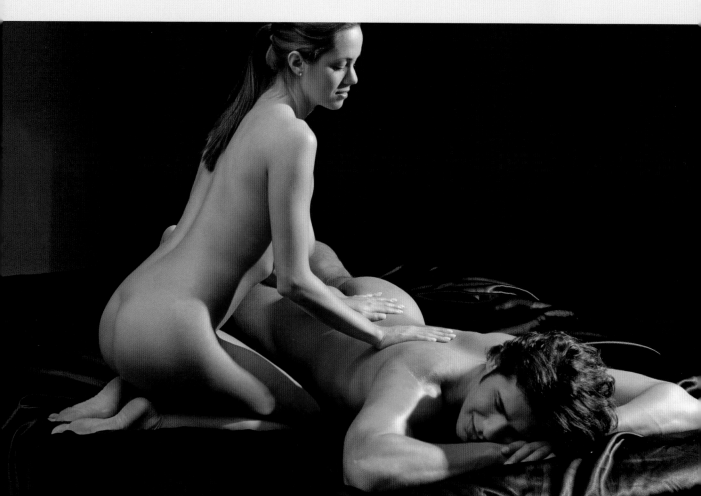

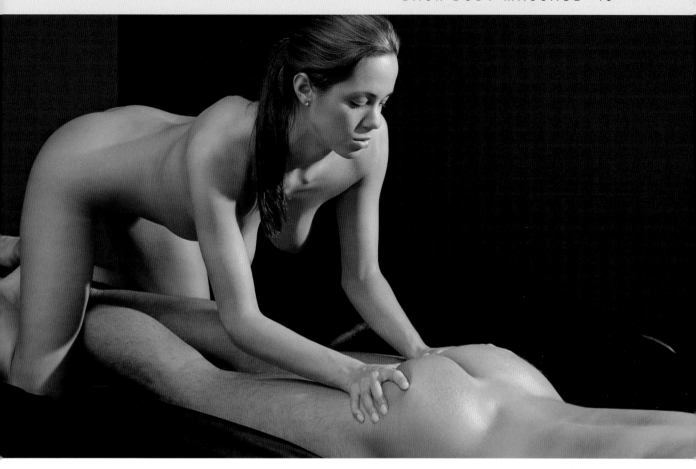

LOWER **BACK BODY** MASSAGE STROKES

Stroke with your whole body to enhance your strength and ease.

Kneeling at his legs, rest a hand on his lower back and pour a tablespoon of massage oil (preferably warm) onto it. Without losing contact with the skin, spread the oil from the buttocks to the bottom of the feet, thereby defining the area you'll be massaging next. In massage, the receiver feels more comfortable knowing what body area will be massaged next. Because unexpected touch surprises and jars the body, introduce each area with light encompassing strokes, then work it in more detail, and conclude with a broad, light finishing stroke. This ritual feels safe and assuring.

Working in more detail now, massage the pads of his feet (similar to the foot-massage strokes in the last chapter). Work your way toward the heart by kneading the calves, either one at a time or simultaneously, by bunching up the muscle in your hands and then releasing it.

Using your whole body as leverage, push your hands firmly up the sensitive inner thigh, up over the buttocks, and back down the outer thigh. Repeat several times. At the point where the leg attaches to the hip (close to the genitals), pull the groin tissue firmly away

from the midline of the body over the sit bones (quite literally the bones under the flesh of the buttocks on which we sit). This move gently massages the genitals without touching them—a subtle hint of pleasure to come.

BUTTOCKS MASSAGE STROKES

Kneeling outside his spread legs, wriggle the butt cheeks, telling your partner to relax his buttocks. Wriggle the fleshy cheeks to your heart's desire. This is pure delight. I guarantee he will not ask you to stop. Any move such as vibrating and jiggling needs to be varied in pressure, tempo, and rhythm, or it becomes repetitive and boring for both the giver and the receiver.

Place a hand at the outside of each cheek and firmly *scoop* your hands toward each other, letting the fleshy cheeks slip out of your grasp as your hands meet over the crack. Go back for another scoop or two. *Knead* the cheeks as a baker kneads bread dough. Check in with him about the pressure of your touch by simply asking a yes-or-no question such as, "Would you like more

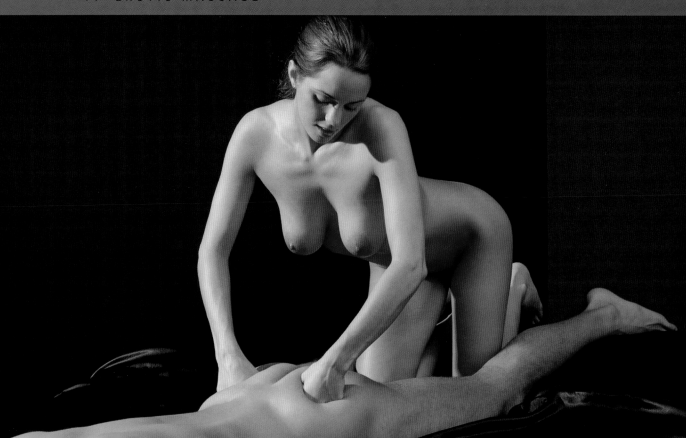

pressure?" You are building trust by inquiring and making adjustments, especially if you don't get defensive. After you adjust your pressure, check in again: "Would you like more pressure?"

Make a fist with your hands and walk them slowly over his buttocks, rotating your wrist as you go. Position your body over your fists in order to use the leverage of your body weight to produce a firm pressure, especially if you are a woman. By letting the weight of your body work for you, you can massage firmly without getting tired or straining the small muscles of your hands and wrists. In addition, you can vary the strokes with lighter pressure throughout the massage.

PERINEUM MASSAGE

The perineum is the area between the scrotum and the anus on a man and the vagina and the anus on a woman. The pelvic-floor muscles in this area are rarely massaged and touch here feels wonderful. We unconsciously hold tension in this area ("tight ass"), and a good perineum massage creates longer and stronger orgasms for both men and women, as well as more ejaculation control for men.

Use the leverage of your body weight to produce a firm pressure.

On a man, the perineum is referred to as the "hidden penis." Almost half of the sensitive, vascular tissue of the penis lies behind the scrotum and inside the pelvis. This "forgotten penis" can be stimulated by a savvy partner for an ecstatic and healthful experience. Usually ignored, the perineum when massaged stimulates the sensitive prostate gland known as the male G-spot, which is both relaxing and exciting. For both sexes, massage to the root or base of the spine vitalizes the sex organs and releases old patterns, inhibitions, and past disappointments, thus creating new opportunity for well-being and intimacy.

Place a flat palm over the perineum with fingers covering the crack and wiggle the hand till you feel the sit bones (close to where the legs meet the pelvis). Place your second hand on top of the first and lean with the weight of your whole body toward the heart. Vibrate and hold. Let the warmth of your presence at his "root" speak silently of your approval of his sexuality. Breathe together. This area can take a great deal of pressure and it translates as feeling secure and loved.

Keeping one hand on the root (the perineum area), slide the other up his back to rest over the heart (left side). Trace this root-to-heart path up and down in several slow strokes varying among vibrating, stillness, rocking, and sounding. Sounding is done by placing your chest over the perineum hand and exhaling your sigh of appreciation, which vibrates his root through your hand. It will help melt the shame we often hold unconsciously at the base of our being.

Kneel beside his left side, or heart side, and place your left hand over his heart area as in the previous heart-sacrum hold. Cup your right hand over the crack with your fingers together on the perineum. Dig the flat full length of your fingers deep into the "hidden penis." Press, rub up and down, massage in circles, vibrate, and hold. Check with him about your pressure. Rock the whole body gently from this firm heart-perineum hold. (Note: On a woman the perineum is much smaller. Do not touch or penetrate the vagina with your hold and rocking. Genital touch will be covered in chapter 6.)

Finish the lower back body massage with several light sweeping strokes in a U shape from the bottom of one foot up the leg, across the sacrum, and down to the other foot.

SLOWNESS IS A DIVINE THING.

We've lost the habit of it. When we move in slow, regular, and harmonious movements, consciousness finds its place. The body begins to enjoy the smallest thing. Attention is heightened. We take in the world full of wonder. We open our senses to the plenitude of sights, sounds, and touch.

Hold, vibrate, and press the perineum toward his heart during a perineum massage.

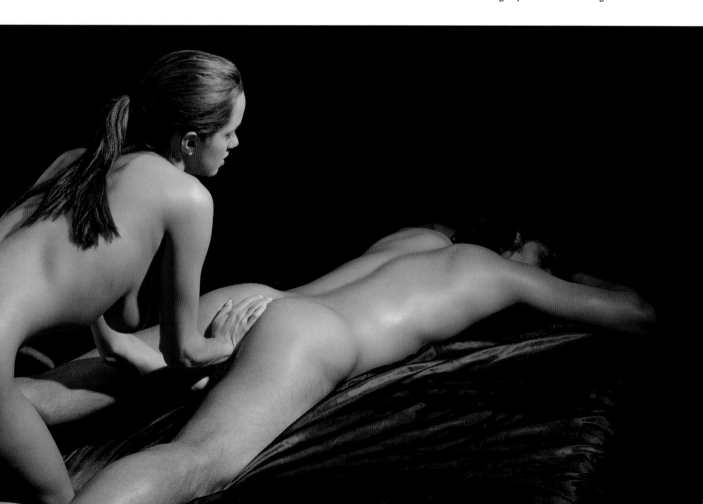

UPPER BACK BODY MASSAGE

Ideally you are about halfway, or ten to fifteen minutes, into your massage. From your kneeling position at his side body, bend down and lay your head and chest on his back, placing an arm over his shoulders and another over his buttocks. Enjoy a back hug. Connect again through the breath and let several vibrating exhales resound through his chest.

Kneeling at his side, rest the back of your hand over his sacrum and put a tablespoon or two of warm oil in the palm. Gently rub your palms together and use both hands to lightly spread the oil with slow, sweeping, broad strokes over the region of the back, shoulders, neck, and arms. You are "introducing" this new upper-back body region with focus, breath, and confidence. You project the thought "You are safe with me; you may let go."

The "opening the seed" stroke
awakens a man's innate playfulness.

OPENING THE SEED GATE

Reach a hand around under the side of the belly at the waist and mirror this movement with the other hand on the opposite side of the belly. Begin a slow, strong pull of the side flesh up and toward the midline of the body. Without lifting your hands away from the body, continue the stroke with each hand around to the opposite belly side. Repeat the pulling-up motion, firmly crisscrossing the back until you have worked up to the shoulders. This motion is called opening the seed gate. When a man wears a belt, the heart center (spontaneity and playfulness) gets disconnected from the genitals (achievement and goal orientation). You are opening a pathway to playful, non-goal-oriented sexuality.

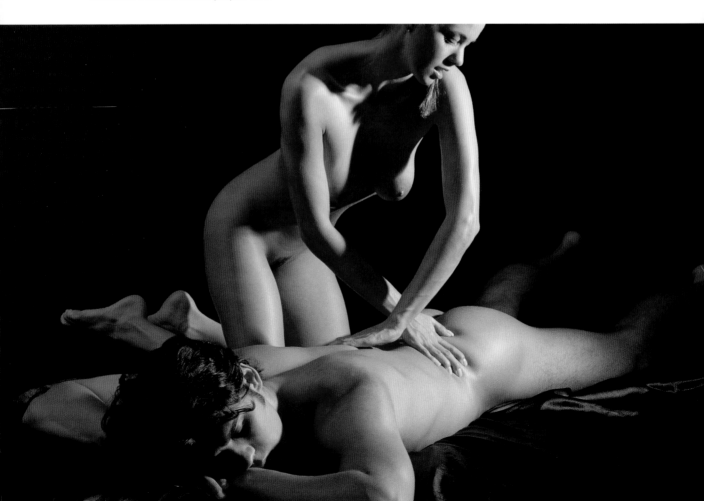

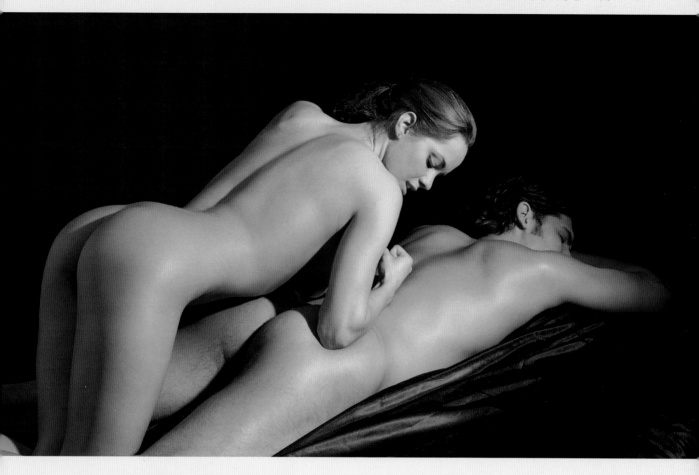

MASSAGE WITH ARMS AND ELBOWS

Positioned between his legs, place the weight of your whole body in your forearms and elbows, and slide them over his back from hip to shoulders, first one side at a time, then both at the same time. Work the buttocks with the elbow right into the hip socket. Ask him, "Do you want less pressure?" Thank him when he responds.

Hover with your weight over your forearms on top of his lung area. Do you feel the pressure of his breath pushing up against your body weight? Ask him to deepen his breath against your steady pressure on the lungs. His breath is as important as your touch in cultivating ecstasy. Coach him into the fullness of the moment by the awesome depth of your own breath.

Use your forearms, elbows, and upper arms to increase the surface area of touch.

Discover the strength and joy of employing bigger-than-hands body parts as massage tools. Use your elbows to come up each side of the spinal column, feeling each vertebra as you go. Use your forearms to come back down the side body under the armpits, squeezing the chest together. Try using the back of your upper arms to pull down the sides of the neck, over the top of the shoulders. Where else can your nonhands body parts fit, jingle, and soothe? Appreciate playing on the rugged territory of the back, but always be gentle with the soft, unprotected area of the kidneys, which are below the ribs and above the waist.

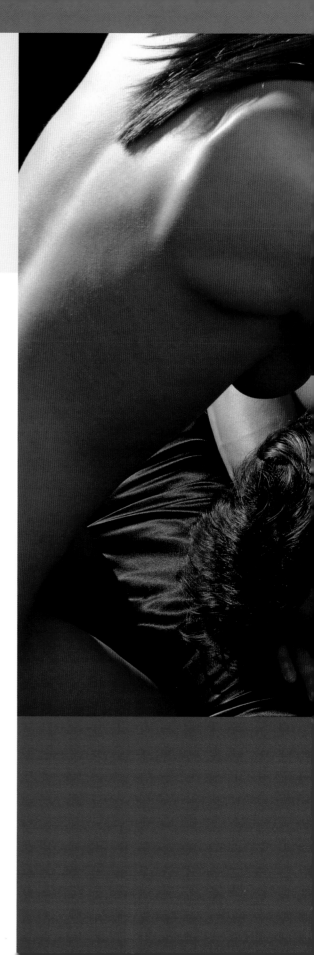

Make all strokes a continuous flow, one blending into another. In a sense, you remember the last stroke and anticipate the next in a continuum. To begin and end a stroke, glide in and off the body. Practice a smooth takeoff and landing. Maintain full hand contact whenever possible.

SHOULDER MASSAGE

Kneeling at his head and facing his feet, place your hands with full contact on his shoulder blades. On an exhale, let your hands slide down the back to his waist, using your body weight behind the stroke. On the inhale, pull up your hands along the sides of the body and over the tips of the shoulders. Repeat this connecting stroke several times, synchronizing your breath with your movement both away from and toward the heart. Move away from the heart on an exhale and toward the heart on an inhale. Try to match your partner's breath.

With the flat pads of your thumbs, make small circles down each side of the spine from the neck to the sacrum. The thumbs mirror each other as they circle outward from the spine. Also, try these same thumb circles around the outer edges of the shoulder blades either one at a time or simultaneously. Vary this stroke by using the palm of the hand.

With the elbows seated in the curve of the shoulders at the base of the neck, lean into the shoulders and vibrate. In one long, smooth stroke, push the shoulders down and out toward the upper arms and reverse back to the neck. Place your thumb in the groove between the shoulder blade and the collarbone and pull outward from the base of the neck to the shoulder tips. Use this stroke on one side at a time, then on both simultaneously.

ARM MASSAGE

Instruct your passive partner to become a rag doll as you choose to move a limb, such as his arm. He is not to help you by lifting it himself. He is in surrender mode; he has turned over his body to you (though he has not lost his voice in the matter if needed). Gently

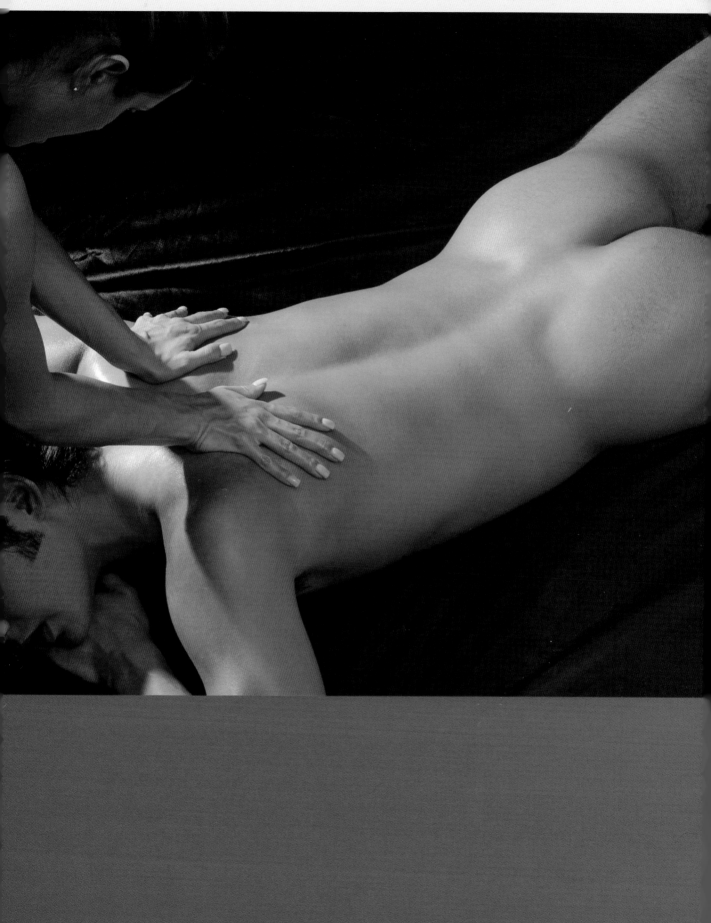

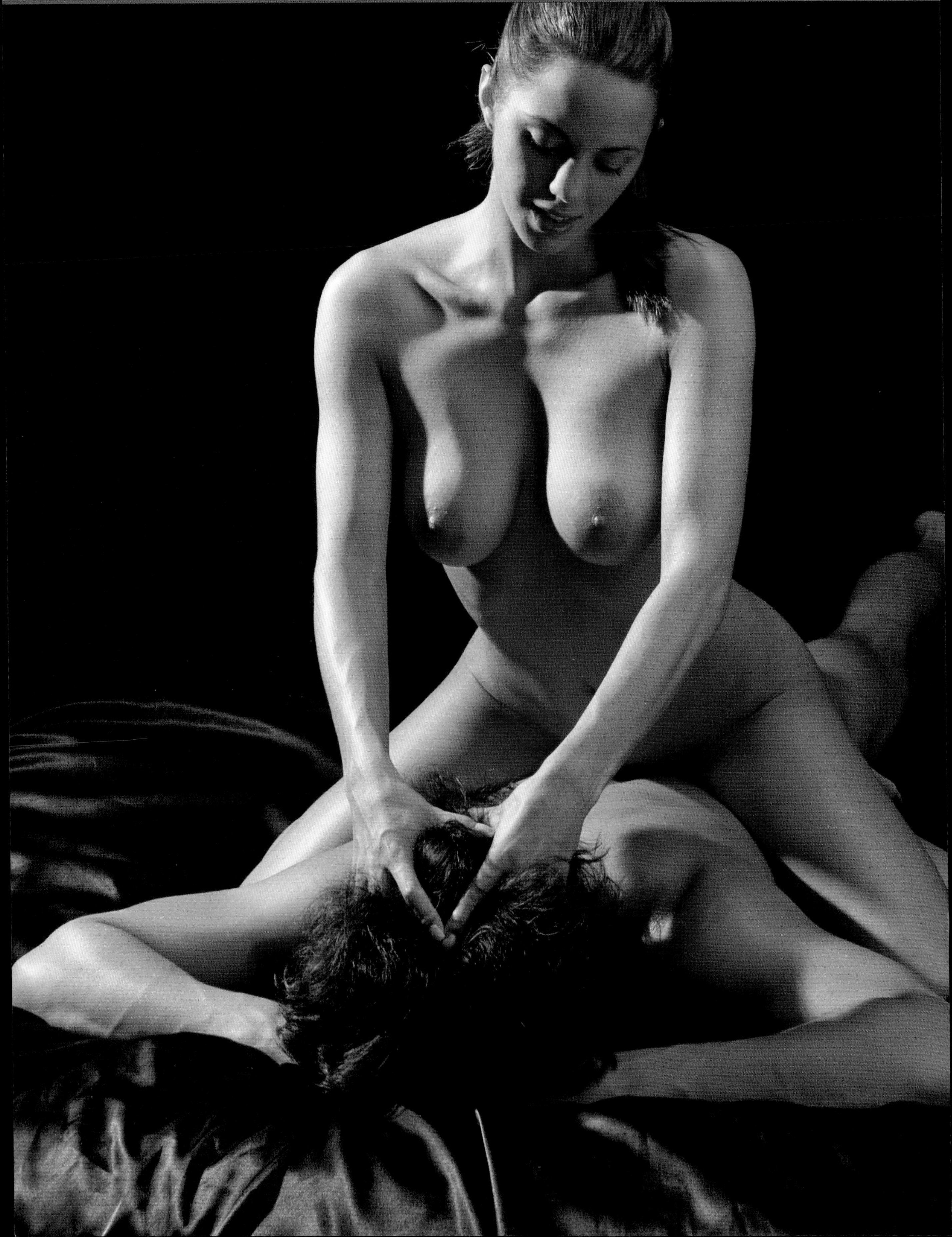

*Breathing with your strokes makes them
more confident, conscious, and powerful.*

lift his arm to test his passive resolve. If it's not limp as
a rag doll, whisper in his ear that you want all of him
like putty in your arms, soft and open.

Holding one or both wrists a few inches above the
bed, gently move his arms around from his sides to over
his head. Wriggle the whole arm. Gently pull the arms
away from the shoulder joints, freeing up any tension
around the joints. Softly shake out the hands.

Laying the arms back down, tug at his fingers.
Cupping a hand over each forearm at the wrist, inhale as
you slide up his arm to the heart in a continuous stroke,
and exhale as you come back down. Repeat this stroke
several times, experimenting with your own variations.
Notice the difference when you breathe with a stroke
and when you do not. Breathing with your strokes
makes them more confident, conscious, and powerful.

NECK AND HEAD
MASSAGE

Massaging the neck and head, we can remember how
often being stuck in the head has interfered with enjoying sensual experiences. We cannot surrender if we are in
our heads. We must learn to let go of analyzing and
simply experience the sensations of touch to enjoy a
massage. If we are comparing a touch with a past experience or thinking about what may happen next, we are
not in the moment (and often feel depressed or anxious).

HEAD MASSAGE STROKES

For the neck and head massage, sit on your partner's
back without too much weight to distract him (or her).
Remind him to follow with his full attention to where
you are touching and when his mind wanders (which is
human nature!), ask him to gently return his full attention to your touch.

Comb your fingers softly through the hair, moving
slowly down closer to the roots and scalp. Rustle his
hair with the pads of your fingers on the scalp, starting
lightly and then more firmly. Catch the hair between
your fingers and pull it until you feel resistance. Ask
him if he wants you to pull harder. Using your finger
pads in circular motions on the scalp, give him a dry
shampoo, really manipulating the tissue between the
hair and the scalp. Don't be too timid here.

Gently tug the soft earlobes downward, pulling the
middle of the ear toward you and the top rim of the
ear upward. Massage the dip behind the ear by the jaw-
bone in a circular motion with your second and third
fingers. Pinch the back of the neck along the vertebrae
between your thumbs and index fingers. Pull up on the
tops of the shoulders where they meet the neck, then
knead in the palm of your hands.

Sensate Focus

The famous sex researchers of the 1960s, William Masters and Virginia Johnson, developed a technique to
help people get out of their heads and into their bodies called sensate focus. Sensate focus encourages each
partner to take turns paying increased attention to their own senses. This method, related to many Tantric
meditative practices from the East, has helped many couples attain high levels of pleasure from massage.

To practice sensate focus, you simply bring your mind's attention to the point of contact on your skin where
you feel you are touching or being touched (both the giver and the receiver perform sensate focus). Whenever
your mind wanders from the touch to other thoughts, you bring it back to the touch sensation points on your
skin. After some time spent on training the mind to focus only on your sensations, you will be able to more easily concentrate, reining in your thoughts when your mind wanders. The results are blissful when the mind stops
chattering and becomes the "slave" of the body in this simple way.

FINISHING
MASSAGE STROKES ON THE BACK BODY

The beauty of erotic massage is celebrating the body as a path to spirit, and celebrating spirit as sensed through the body. In the West, we have not celebrated the connection between spirituality and sexuality that was prevalent for thousands of years in ancient Taoist, Hindu, and Buddhist teachings. In our dualistic view of good and bad, right and wrong, we delegate spirit as divine and fear the flesh as something distracting us from the divine. No wonder reclaiming our body as a pathway to the divine is so powerful.

The body is the earthly temple for the soul and deserves our reverence. Say good-bye to the back body with the same full-body sweeping strokes you used to introduce the massage coming into the body. Kneeling at his side, stroke him from head to foot with both hands in a long, continuous path down each side of the body. Using a light touch, be aware in your mind of connecting all the parts of the body into one integrated whole being. Sense all of his body at once with your touch. Include the shoulders, arms, and hands as you trace the whole body.

You may wish to do finishing strokes with a peacock feather or by floating a silk scarf over him. Make each brush of the feather be like a prayer honoring him as an aspect of the divine. Make your last stroke as intentional as your first. I like to finish with gently resting my hands over the heart and sacrum and then lifting them off slowly, almost imperceptibly. After you release your last touch, rest in stillness next to him, simply holding space for him to absorb your appreciation. Wait till he moves and then offer a heart salutation or melting hug. You may even choose to spoon together in silence.

When you are ready, you may wish to talk about the experience. How did your intention help guide your surrender or experience? What did your partner do that particularly encouraged your letting go? Did you feel you could communicate your deep feelings or needs to the giver? How did tuning in to and slowing the breath work or not work?

Instead of minimizing talking as you did on this massage, another time you may want to talk about the strokes as you massage. Silence helps you center and surrender, but coaching your partner about what you like is a great way to improve your skills. Occasionally a verbal massage works wonders. You can also reverse the order of the massage and start with the head and end with the feet.

"I was so relaxed as my girlfriend lightly brushed my back with a feather that I think I fell asleep. She must have kept touching me, because I had incredibly euphoric sensations as I drifted in and out. She made me feel like anything I did was okay, so I didn't have to worry about responding. I loved it. It was so freeing."

—Jonathan, 28

The body is the temple of the soul. Honoring the back body with the light brush of a feather can be both a sensual and soul-enriching experience.

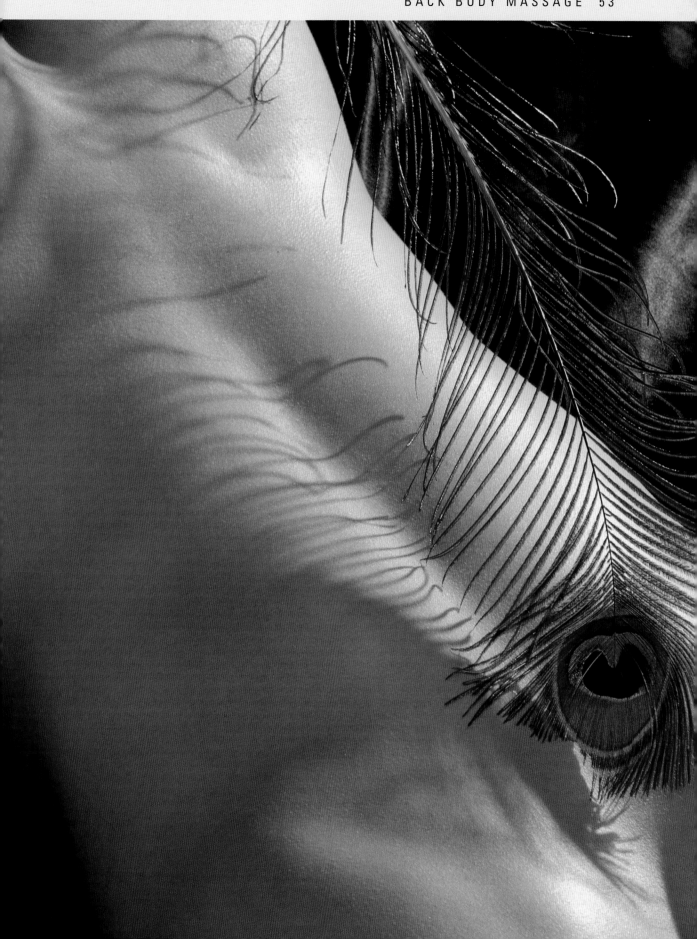

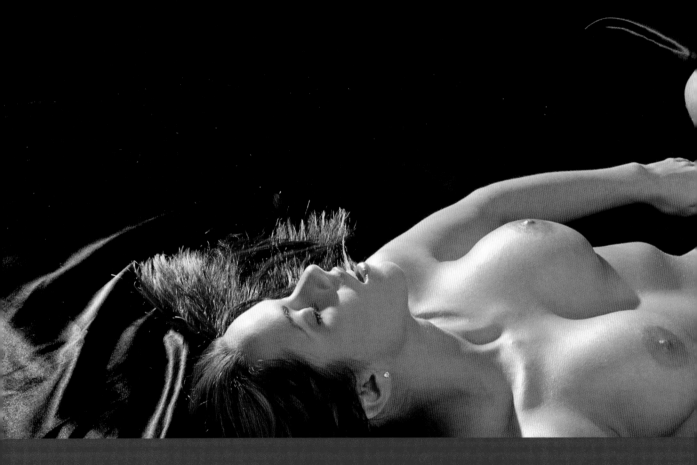

chapter
FOUR

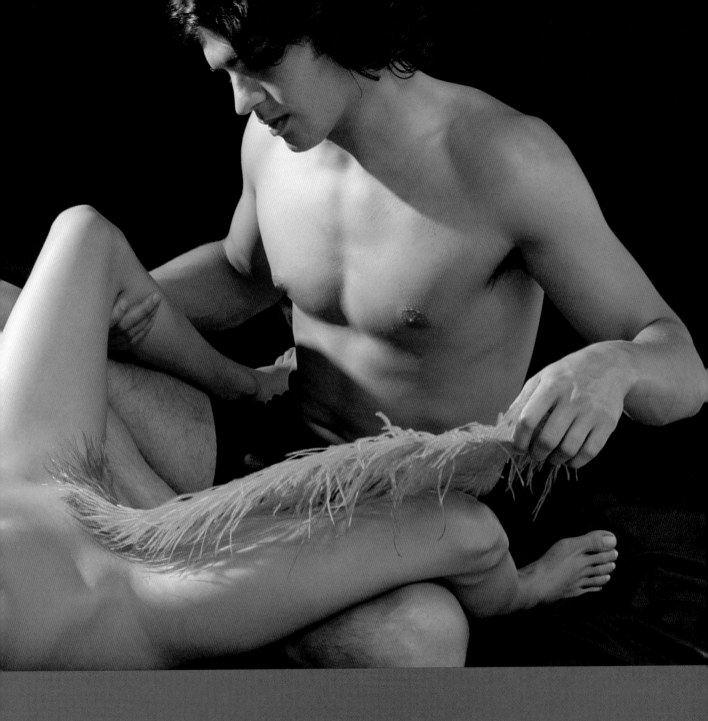

EROTIC FRONT BODY MASSAGE

LOVING OUR BODIES

The back body was a perfect place to practice deep surrender, whereas the front body brings up new challenges that may interfere with enjoying an erotic massage. All of us have issues with our bodies. We all wish they looked different. When we are worried about how our partner may view our body, we lose the joy of being in the moment and sensing his touch. Being massaged on the front body, with our breasts and genitals exposed, we feel particularly vulnerable.

BODY IMAGE

All of us have been told, or have somehow come to the conclusion, that our body isn't "right." This or that part droops, is too small, too flabby, too freckly—and the list goes on and on. These negative messages stay with us (generally for a long time, if not forever!) and can translate into our not wanting to be touched there and can even dull our sensations. Aging bodies challenge our grace and acceptance of ourselves. Can we learn to see added weight, wrinkles, and a receding hairline not as imperfections but as measures of experience and wisdom?

Becoming more comfortable, accepting, and appreciative of your body will increase the pleasure you can receive from the massages that follow in this book. To deepen your enjoyment of sensual touch, start by revealing the naked truth about your body to yourself and your partner and loving it. These body-image exercises can break down your barriers to intimacy, increase your pleasure, and bring amazing closeness with your partner.

Body-Image Mirror: Solo Exercise

Take time by yourself (at least fifteen minutes) to stand completely naked in front of a full-length mirror to evaluate and rediscover your body in detail. This may seem strange or difficult, but alone time with your nakedness, with the intention of fostering compassion and support for your body, is fundamental to enjoying it with another person.

Undress and take an inventory of your entire body. Be like an outsider looking on and evaluate every part as an objective observer. Start at the top of your head and, talking aloud, comment on your hair. What color and texture is it? What do you like/dislike about it? Move to your hairline, then your forehead. Describe in detail each of your features—eyes, nose, and cheekbones. How do you feel about each part? Don't get sidetracked by a new wrinkle or mole. Comment out loud as you move down the body, candidly observing your neck, shoulders, breast, abdomen, and genitals. Turn around and, looking over your shoulder, comment on your back body.

Be honest and say what you like about your body, even though it feels wrong or narcissistic to compliment yourself. You can say aloud, "My skin tone is creamy and my shoulders are square and strong-looking." Can you appreciate how your life experiences have uniquely distinguished your body? Can you accept how life is being "worn" on your body? After you have gone all the way down to the toes, encourage self-compassion toward this divinely crafted, one-of-a-kind body. End by acknowledging your body temple in the mirror with a reverent heart salutation.

"I said things about my body that I had previously only thought to myself, but somehow hearing my voice softened my criticism. I almost started laughing at some of my complaints, and then a strange thing happened. I saw a body in the mirror that had accompanied me on every step of my journey in life, and I began to cry. In that body I experienced all the pain, sadness, excitement, and joy I'd ever known, and I was so grateful."

—Amanda, 39

Body-Image Mutual Exercise

Now it is time to share a body-image exercise with your partner. Rarely do we get the opportunity to really look at another person's naked body. We usually "sneak" quick glances at breasts or genitals, but now we give permission to really look at each other's nakedness. You may feel awkward at first, even if you have been with this person a long time, but consenting to see each other in your most natural state with awareness and intention is an amazingly intimate and vulnerable exercise.

Set aside at least fifteen minutes with your partner. Undress and stand nude in front of each other, about arm's length apart or whatever spatial distance feels comfortable. Close your eyes, tune in to your partner's breathing, and find your rhythm together. When you feel the harmony of shared breathing, without conversation, open your eyes and, beginning at your partner's hairline, observe every detail of his or her body. Move to the forehead, then look deep into each other's eyes. You are seeing with the eyes of a child before being told that staring is rude.

Move gradually and silently down the face, then from one area to the next on the body. Take a deliberate, long look at the breasts, belly, and pubic area. Stare until you have had enough and you feel any charge of shame or discomfort dispelled. Turn around one at a time to observe the back of your partner's body. Take in every scar, vein, mole, and pore. Without talking, view each other all the way down to the toes with curiosity and openness, and without judgment. *See beyond your nakedness and into each other's souls.* End with a heart salutation and a long hug.

Body-Image Mirror: Partner Exercise

In this last body-image exercise, you will repeat the first exercise, but this time with your partner. Allow about twenty minutes for each person and decide who will first be active. In front of a full-length mirror, the active partner stands and evaluates his entire body, talking out loud as if there were no one else in the room, while the passive partner sits silently behind him. Starting at the head, describe the color and texture of your hair. Do you like the shape of your ears? What do you think about your brow, eyebrows, and each facial feature? Talk about your neck, shoulders, chest, and breast. You are noticing, revealing, and exposing your true feeling about each part.

If a memory or story comes up, feel free to speak it. Touch your body as you talk, if you like. How did it feel to grow up in this body? When did you first discover your genitals? What messages did you get growing up with these male or female sex organs? What body parts bring you pleasure; what parts bring you pain? How have you matured with this body? Are you good friends with your body or are you at odds?

If you are the passive partner, you might notice if your lover leaves out some body part or feature. You may wonder why it was forgotten. We need to accept the unloved or shameful parts of us if we are to become whole. You may choose to later ask your partner about any omissions. In your massage, vow to specially love and honor any unloved parts. Appreciate how vulnerable your partner is in disclosing his deepest feelings, fears, and shortcomings about his body. End with a heart salutation, then reverse roles.

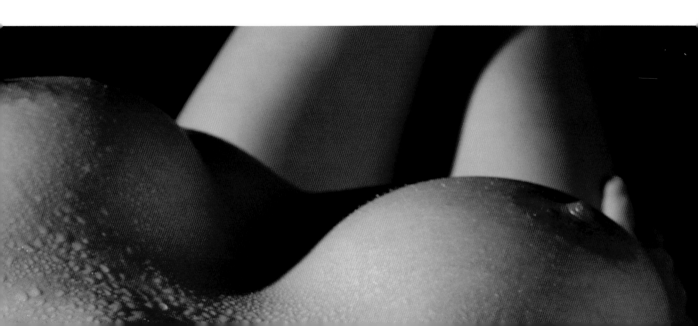

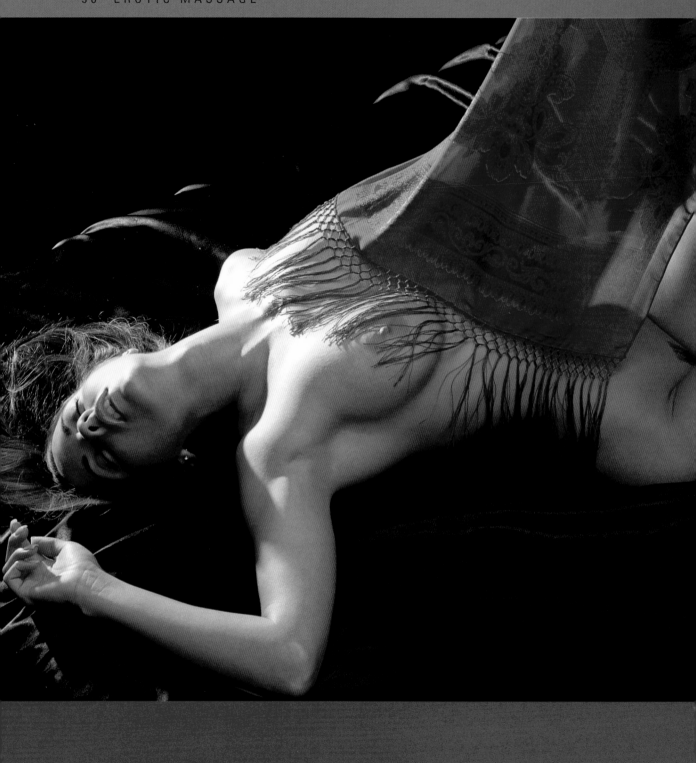

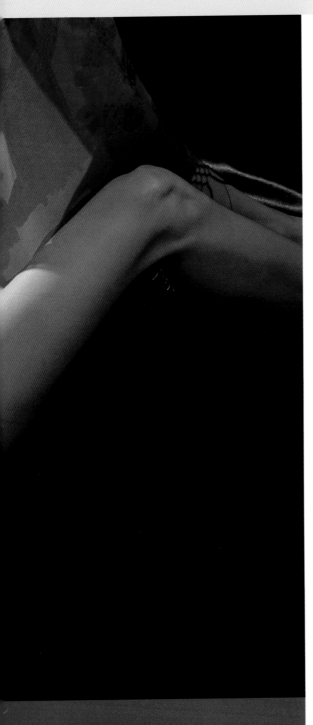

Float a silk scarf over your lover's body, allowing the fringe to tickle her inner thighs.

COMING INTO THE
BODY

Tell your passive partner (the woman this time) that she deserves some luscious time to receive a front body massage, and you have set aside twenty to thirty minutes to pamper her body. Remind her to relax, breathe deeply, and in the spirit of sensate focus, be mindful only of your touch. A good intention for you both would be, "To follow every touch with every breath."

Sit at her left side, the heart side, and softly rest your right hand on her heart and your left hand over the pubic mound. Imagine a woman's energy flowing down from the heart into the genitals (whereas a man's energy flow is reversed, flowing from his genitals to his heart). Gaze into each other's eyes and breathe together till you feel a connection. Remember, this is the first time in the massage sequence that genitals are exposed. Approve of her body, voicing affirmations such as, "This body brings me so much pleasure. What a gift to me."

Choose among the following ideas for a soft introduction to touching the front body.

• Silk scarf
Orchestrate your opening moves soothingly. Float a silk scarf over the length of her body. Remember, lighter and slower; less is more. Let the fringe tickle her inner thighs. Come up from the feet with the scarf, gently pulling it up between her legs and over her genitals. Whisper to her, "I adore you. I cherish you. I love you."

• Rabbit fur
You may choose to put on your chinchilla or rabbit-fur mitt and stroke her head to toe. See how slow and continuous your moves can be. You are teasing her, and women never get enough of it. Slide the mitt between the toes, between her fingers, and with just the fur, touch her nipples, face, and ears.

• Cornstarch powder

You may wish to try what I call the "angel touch." Rub about a teaspoon of cornstarch powder (yes, from your kitchen!) between your hands and surprise her with the silkiest touch experience yet. Lightly spread with full-hand contact the powder up and down one entire side of the body, then repeat on the other side. If her eyes are closed, she'll wonder how your touch got so heavenly. She'll marvel at your sensuality.

• Feather

Move to sit cross-legged at her feet, pulling her legs over your thighs and, with a feather (or feather duster), make several long U strokes, starting at one foot, going up the inner leg, over the pubic mound, and down to the other foot. Include a stroke or two that go up to the heart and breasts. From this position, you can blow a long, cool, steady stream of air on her genitals.

• Vibrator

If you have a vibrator, cup your hand with your palm over her genitalia. Place the vibrator against the back of your hand. The vibrations coming through your hand will be gentle and teasing, stirring the imagination for later play. Since the front massage includes genitals without solely focusing on them, she has the opportunity to cultivate desire and contain excitement for you. Often this opportunity is missing for women, since men are so much quicker in their excitement and desire to move straight to the genitals.

COACH HER BREATHING

Keep your palm over the genitals (without a vibrator) and place your other hand gently over her abdomen. As the giver, you are also the breath coach. All your great touching will be of little consequence unless her deep breathing focuses her mind and carries her into the bliss of the moment.

Synchronize your breath with your lover's—in and out together—bringing you into greater intimacy. If her breathing is inaudible, and you are unable to distinguish her inhale or exhale, whisper to her, "I'm lost; where are you in the breath?" Once your breathing is synchronized, rest your hand on her pubic mound. Keep the hand still on the inhale, and vibrate it gently on your shared exhale.

COACH HER SOUNDING

As her breathing coach, make audible sighs and sounds on your exhale to encourage her to let go and vibrate with you. Loosen your throat and let the sound out without effort. If you are not self-conscious about making noise, your partner is more likely to follow. Encourage her sounding by saying, "It's so sexy to hear your breath. I love to hear your sounds; thank you." Imagine with your vibrations that all your inhibitions (and hers) are shaking loose and falling away. *Imagine on the exhale that your sound is filling her up, penetrating her with your desire for closeness.*

We have much resistance to making sound, even in lovemaking. We've been taught to be quiet breathers, quiet about our desires, and quiet about our passions. Quiet may be fine for therapeutic massage, but not for erotic massage. Rebel against the silence. Breathe big, breathe loud. Merge your sighs with your lover's. *Breathing and sounding—these are the body's tools for ecstasy.* Use them, expand them. If necessary, give each other permission to fake it until you make it.

Make several long U strokes when caressing your partner with a feather. Encourage her to breathe evenly and slowly, sighing on the exhale.

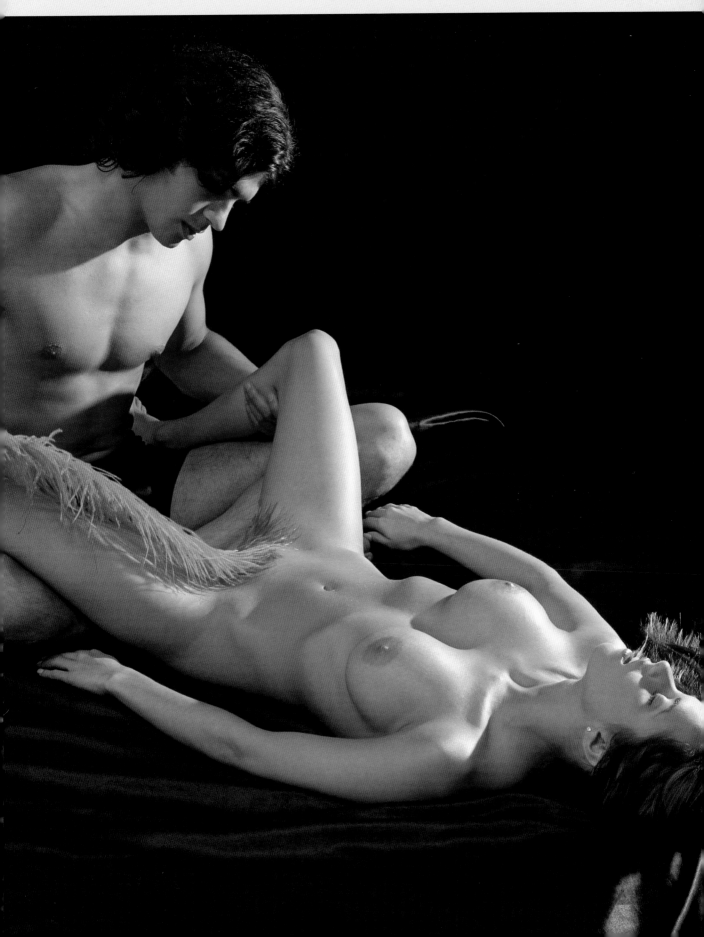

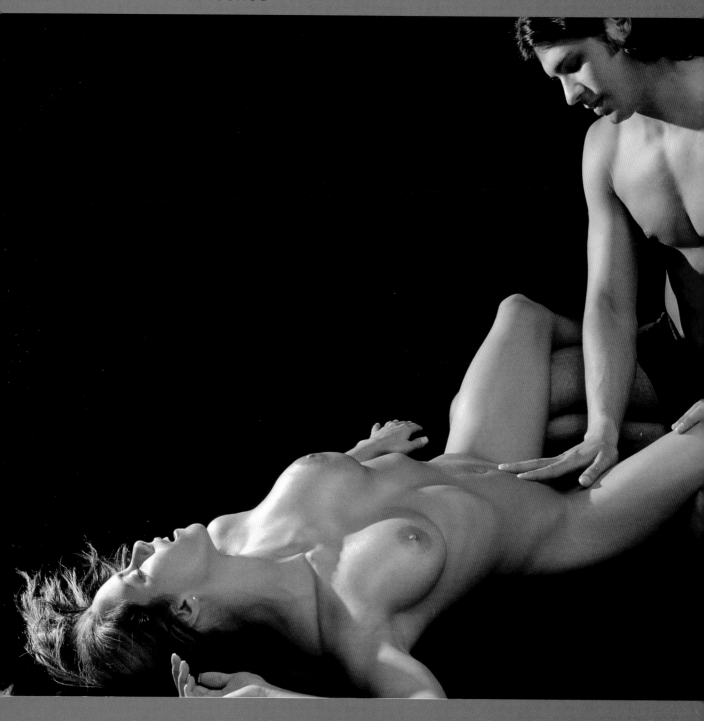

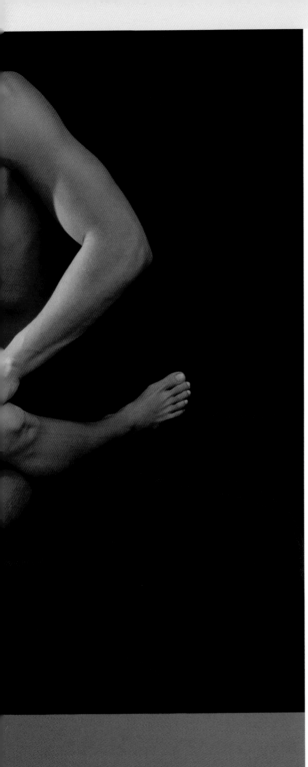

The sensation of one palm resting on the abdomen while the other hand moves over the body feels assuring and protective to the receiver.

LOWER FRONT
BODY MASSAGE

You have awakened her body lusciously with silks, furs, or feathers. You have coached her breath and sound into deeper surrender, and now you will go deeper with your strokes. Sit between her legs and pull her knees over your thighs. Pour some warm oil into your hand and reverently spread it over her legs, feet, and abdomen.

THE U STROKE

Rest your right palm on the pubic bone with the fingers pointing toward the navel. With the left hand, stroke down the right leg to the foot and back in a continuous movement. Replace the right hand resting on the pubic bone with the left hand in a smooth and imperceptible transfer, then progress down the left leg with the right hand. Repeat several times, making the transition smoothly and confidently. Always keep one hand covering the pubic mound; it feels assuring and protective. Vary the stroke by progressing up to include the heart center between the breasts before transferring hands on the lower abdomen.

"At first, breathing and making sounds was embarrassing for me, but I was determined to try it and told my partner of my desire to experiment. That was several months ago. Now, I can't imagine trying to go to the places I go to during a massage with a normal breath. I'm on a whole other level now. Breathing deeply got me there."
—David, 31

WEAK IN THE KNEES

In mapping the body's pleasure zones, don't forget the back of the knees. Gently raise her leg over your shoulder and tease under her thigh and knee with your fingertips or the back of your hand. Most women love a man to come close to the genitals and then back away. Remember the general rule: If there are two of them (knees, thighs, etc.), do them both.

Tease is frequently the forgotten element of female arousal. Women often feel rushed to climax. It is men's nature to want to please a woman, to "produce" for her. The man should move leisurely and take the time to entice his lover. Cultivate greater depth of consciousness in your touching; be the container for her budding ecstasy by staying present to your touch.

"I love it when he comes close to my lotus flower and then moves away without touching. I feel his imaginary fingers playing and I build desire for him."

—Melinda, 43

Women often feel rushed to climax, so men should not forget about teasing. Gently raise her leg over your shoulder and tease under her thigh and knee with your fingertips or the back of your hand.

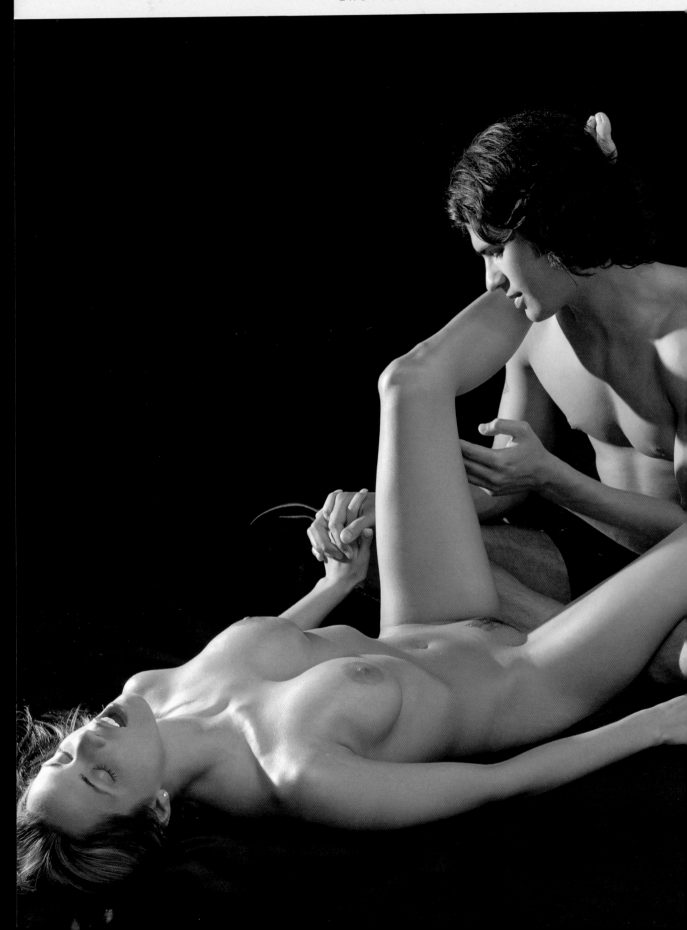

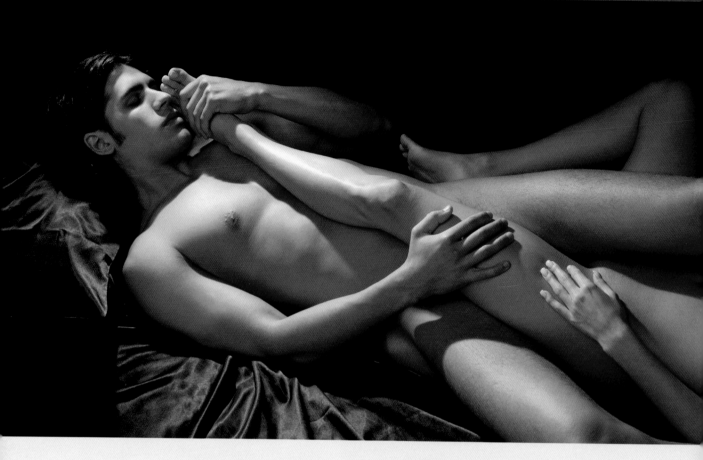

ALTERNATING-LEG MASSAGE

Lean back to a supine position and pull her leg up between yours till the foot is close to your face. From this scissors position you can easily massage her feet, calves, and thighs. Be aware that in your role as giver, as in receiving, you are to focus only on your sensations. Feel the weight of her leg on your chest. Take time to notice the heat of it on your body. Feel her leg rise on your chest with your breath and lower with your exhale. Be sure to change legs and perform the same movements.

Press both thumbs into the sole of the foot above the heel and knead in small circles. Continue the circles up to the pad of the foot. Slide a finger in and out between the toes, then pinch and rub the webbing between the toes with your thumb and index finger. Breathe into the very point where your skin touches hers. When your attention wanders off on some thought, acknowledge it, smile, then return your thoughts to the moment and to the touch. Our minds are relieved to know they don't have to do everything. They can sit back and enjoy the ride sometimes. How refreshing for the mind to simply observe the wonder and delight of the feeling body.

To finish the lower body, kneel between her legs and, facing her, pull her thighs up over yours. Stroke broadly from foot to foot over the abdomen in several sweeping U strokes.

Massage the feet, calves, and thighs in the scissor position.

"Because I'm a nurse, I'm on my feet most of the day. There is nothing I relish more than when my husband gives me a leg and foot massage when I get home from work. Sometimes he tenderly undresses me for it and feathers me under the knee. It brings me to a Zen sort of space. We'll end kissing and sometimes have sex right there. Other times we linger in that prolonged orgasmic realm and end up smiling like starstruck lovers over dinner. Going to bed with him on those nights is magical."

—Sarah, 34

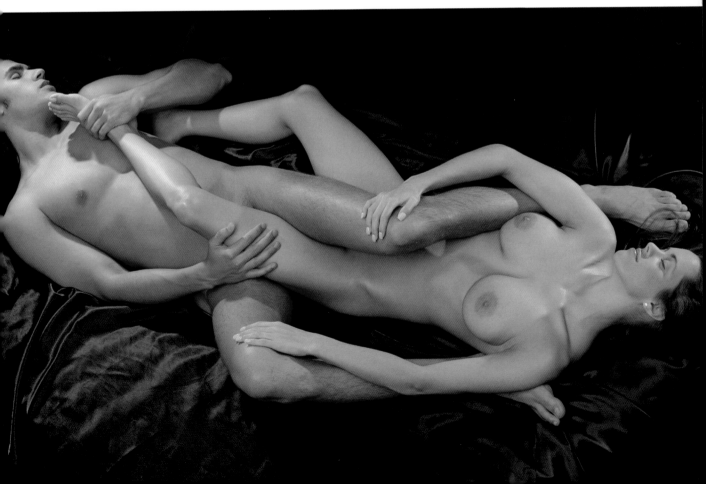

UPPER FRONT
BODY MASSAGE

From your kneeling position between her legs, rub oil over her upper body, starting with the abdomen, coming up between the breasts with one hand following the other. At the collarbone, press outward toward the tips of the shoulders, then stroke down the arms all the way to the fingertips, where you will lift gently off. Repeat this sweeping introductory stroke a few times, then casually circle some oil around the breasts, without focusing on the nipple.

• Abdomen
With a clockwise motion, circle the navel with one or two flat hands, covering an area about the size of a dinner plate. Be gentle with the belly. Feel the ridge of the lower ribs and outline it with your flat fingertips. If you circle using two hands, one will gently slide over the other without breaking the stroke. Slide both hands up the side body from the hips, lifting up the outside tissue of the breast as you reach the underarm.

• Shoulders, Arms, and Hands
Place both palms on the upper chest, above the breasts, with your fingers pointing to the ten-o'clock and two-o'clock positions; firmly press outward toward the shoulder tips. Slide your fingers along the underside of the collarbone, working from the neck outward and back again several times. Knead the upper shoulders and arms by manipulating the musculature between your thumb and fingers, moving downward to the forearms and wrists. Encourage her to go limp, like a rag doll, as you lift her wrists and massage them, and shake out the hands and limp fingers. Squeeze her palms, separating the finger pads, and gently tug her fingertips away from the body.

• Breast Massage
Women love to have their breasts massaged, particularly if the man doesn't act too eager to get there. You have taken time to massage and caress the whole body, which women crave, and now it's time for a special treat.

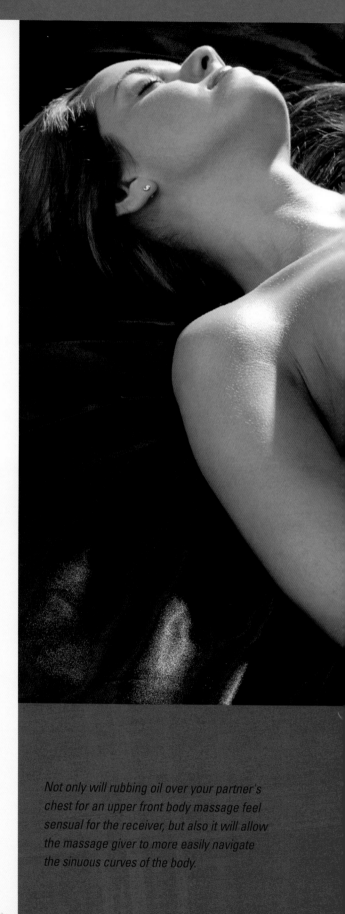

Not only will rubbing oil over your partner's chest for an upper front body massage feel sensual for the receiver, but also it will allow the massage giver to more easily navigate the sinuous curves of the body.

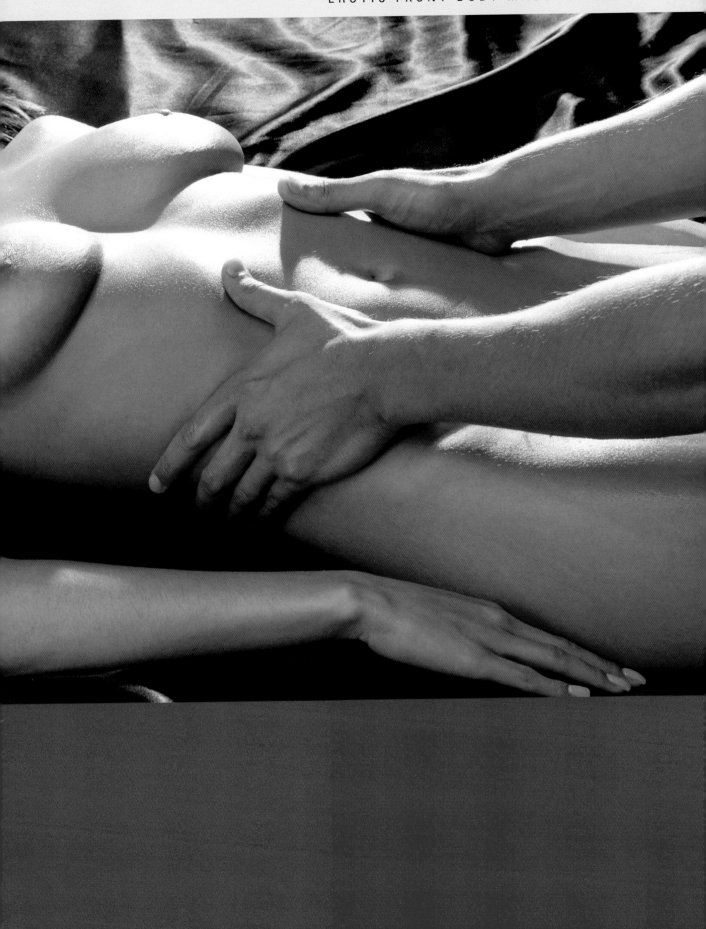

Some women report a direct zing right from the breast through the core of the body to the genitals. Men, as well as women, can enjoy breast stimulation. If a man thinks only women enjoy being touched in this erogenous zone, it will be harder for him to notice the gentle sensations of this area. Many men have experienced increased nipple sensation by simply allowing themselves the pleasure.

Lesbians are well practiced in how to draw out and prolong the pleasure of breast stimulation. Studies show that they spend a much longer time in this area than most heterosexual couples. The breasts emanate heart energy and represent, especially in a woman, her desire to nurture and give to others. By massaging your lover's breasts, you are replenishing her well of caring emotion that is likely to come right back to you in a loving river.

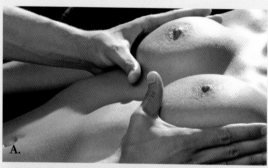

A.

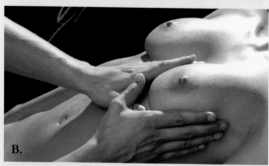

B.

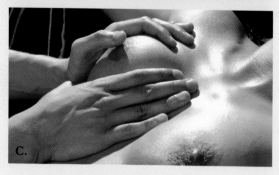

C.

Breast Massage Strokes

Kneeling between her legs or sitting at her side, add more oil to your hands and, cupping a hand around each breast, vibrate the fleshy tissue. Scoop as much of the breast tissue as possible and gently wiggle your hands. Tell her how beautiful her breasts are and how much pleasure it brings you to touch them. Most women think they are too big, too small, or too something. Support her surrender in this vulnerable area with your deep breathing and conscious touch. If she feels you are trying to "perform" for her, she'll feel the need to "respond" to you instead of focusing on her own pleasure.

A. Place a hand on the outside of each breast, under her arms, and scoop up the outside breast tissue until it slides out from under your hands. This feels delightful. Try this stroke vibrating. Massage in a firm circular movement the dip between the shoulder tips and the breasts. Vibrate the breast tissue from this ten-o'clock and two-o'clock position.

B. With both hands on one breast, encircle the entire breast, gently pulling up on it and squeezing. Using your fingertips, press small circles in a large circular pattern around the entire breast. Cup both hands over one breast and take the time to feel its silky texture and softness. Gently squeeze your hands together, kneading the tissue in a circular movement. Stay with soft, broad movements and avoid singling out the nipple. Ask her about the pressure. Repeat these movements on the other breast.

C. Experiment with tracing patterns such as a *spiral* up to the nipple and back. Come into the nipple like a spider web with five fingers spread out and coming to one point at the nipple. Use a light touch at first. If nipples are touched too hard at the beginning, she may put up a barrier for fear of being touched too hard too fast.

"I love it when my husband rubs oil on my breasts. He knows how sensitive they are, and scoops, vibrates, and massages them perfectly. When he plays with my nipple I feel both relaxed and sexually energized at the same time"

—Lynn, 40

Only now are you ready to play with the nipple, the most sensitive part. Cupping the entire breast tissue with your hands, use your thumb to barely brush over the oiled tip of the nipple. Pause. Breathe. Go back and teasingly flick the nipple with your thumb. Stop moving. Silence is a stroke. Come in again and rotate the nipple at the end of your thumb. Pause. Err on the side of too little, not too much.

Lick the nipple lightly. Blow cool air on it. No mouth mauling. Come in to where she can feel your hot breath just hanging over the nipple. Breathe several deep breaths without touching, just breath on skin. If you leave her wanting more, you've done your job.

HEAD MASSAGE

You may wish to have her head in your lap for these strokes. Comb your fingers lavishly through her hair, gathering it into large clumps in your hands and gently tugging. Firmly massage the scalp in small circles with your finger pads, feeling the scalp move over the head bones. With your thumbs, make small circles at her temples and behind her jaw.

With all eight of your fingertips, find the ridge where the skull meets the neck. Holding the weight of her head a couple of inches off your lap, knead this ridge with your fingertips. Gently rotate her head in both hands (remind her to assume rag-doll mode) and move it in a clockwise motion, pausing and holding at the top where the chin moves toward the breastbone.

Letting someone move your head is a supreme gesture of surrender and trust. Start slowly and check with your receiver to find out how far feels comfortable. If you feel safe, someone moving a body part for you can be euphoric.

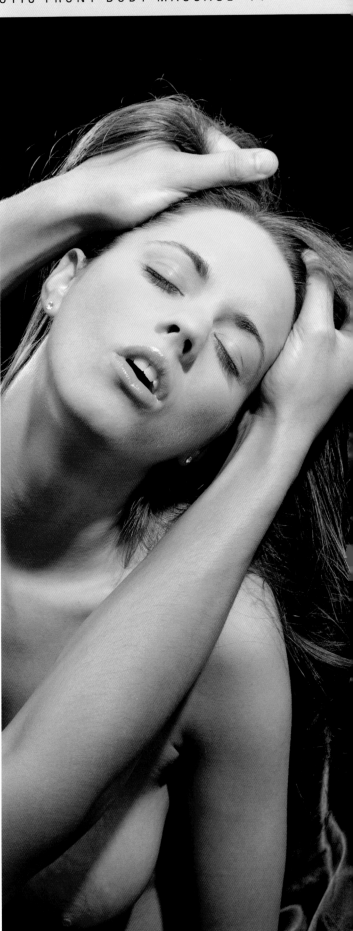

FINISHING STROKES
FOR THE FRONT BODY

Lie next to your beloved. Place your hand over her heart. Think of penetrating her heart with your caring, your protection, and your love. Breathe together with eyes open or closed. Brush your fingertips lightly over as much of her body as you can comfortably reach, connecting her body parts. You may choose to cover her with a sheet or a blanket and leave her to soak in the afterglow of your kindness. You may both decide to do the relaxation bonding (discussed in chapter 2) —spooning and holding. You may choose to continue with a genital massage or even the sexual bonding exercise (chapter 8).

If you do not get to all of these strokes in the twenty-to-thirty-minute front massage it just means you have more to explore (and invent) the next time. You can also renegotiate a longer time frame with your partner. Assuming a change in plan, though, without checking with your lover is not advisable. You build trust and safety by honoring your commitments, such as the time frame.

Massage and Trust

Trust *is strengthened by staying within the boundary of the massage—for example, not fondling the genitals on a front massage. Many men have lamented to me in my sex-coaching practice that their partners no longer want to be massaged. Upon my inquiry, often it's revealed that massage as foreplay for sex is what they were really offering. Successful sensual massage demands the highest integrity. Clearly express your desires and intentions and listen mindfully; massage should be consensual, not manipulative.*

Massage is a natural lead into sexual play and being spontaneous is the beauty of being in the moment. So there may be times when you both *spontaneously choose to change the boundaries. Playfulness will grow naturally out of a foundation of trust where boundaries have been repeatedly respected in the past.*

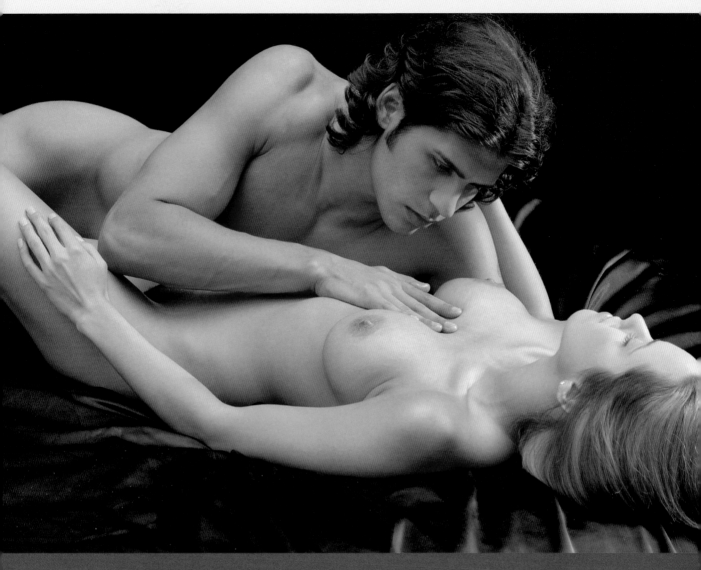

Surrender your mind, breath, and body;
let your lover penetrate you with his heart.

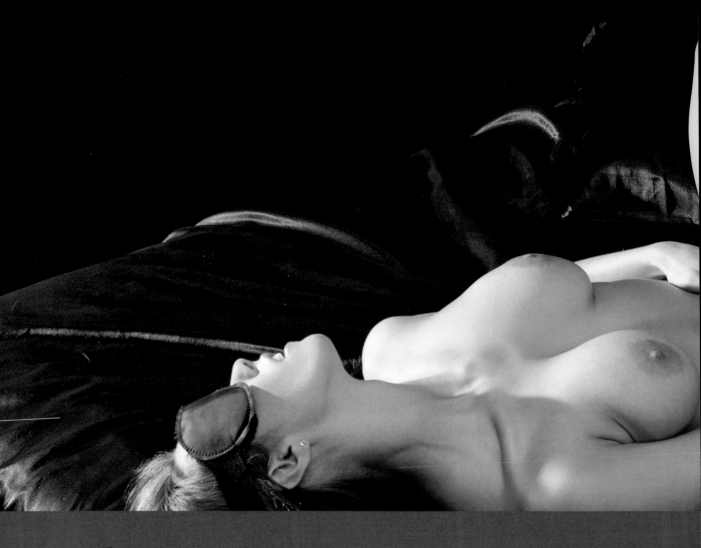

chapter

FIVE

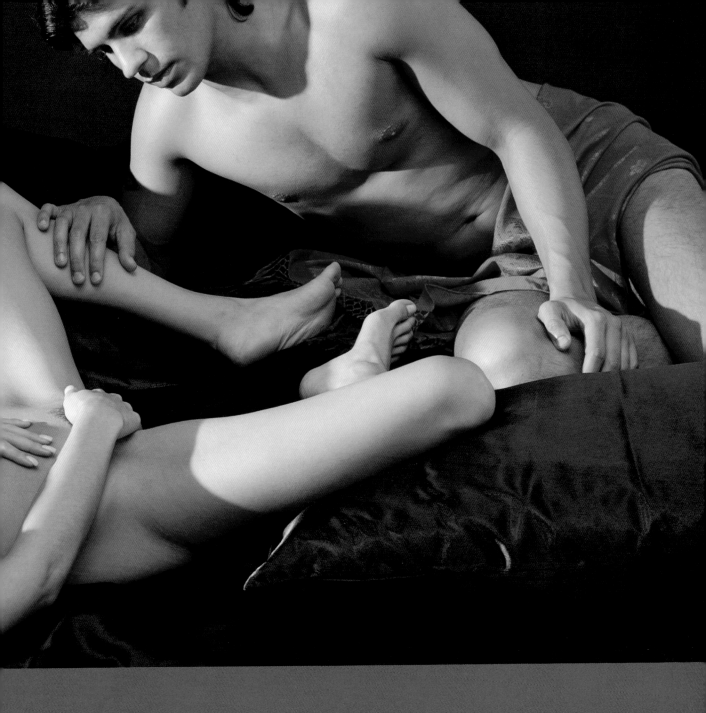

EROTIC SELF-MASSAGE

If you were asked who your first lover was, you probably wouldn't respond, "Myself," though most likely discovering your genitals was first done by you. Masturbation is the most prevalent of all sexual acts, yet it is often veiled in shame and guilt. Growing up, most of us were probably not taught that touching ourselves is a natural and healthy expression. We grew up hiding our solo sexuality, masturbating silently and quickly (not to get caught). Today most of our self-pleasuring is still affected by those early hidden experiences that inhibit our sexual creativity and growth.

Changing the way you touch yourself translates into changing the way you touch your partner. If you no longer masturbate to get the job done, relieve stress, or use it as a sleeping pill, you are free to explore self-loving as a creative, evolving erotic expression. The exercises in this chapter lay the foundation to enhanced partner genital massage by first expanding your self-loving potential.

WOMAN'S EROTIC SELF-MASSAGE RITUAL

The attitude you bring to pleasing yourself speaks directly to how you feel about pleasing your partner. Choose to bring more pleasure and fun into your life by planning a special self-pleasuring session. Call a girlfriend or a lover and tell him that you are making a solo loving date with yourself. Pamper yourself by buying some special gift that day to add to the enjoyment of your evening home alone.

SELF-TOUCH PREPARATION FOR WOMEN

Prepare your sacred, sexy space with candles, scents, music, and any "props," such as costumes, boas, lingerie, oils, lotions, and sex toys. Prepare a bath with scented salts and bubbles. Let your housemates or family know you'd like privacy and put a "Do not disturb" sign on the door. Call your friend or lover (who also may be treating himself to a self-loving ritual at the same time!) and let him know you are beginning your one-hour self-loving session. Now turn off your phone and focus only on your pleasure for the next hour.

Often we think someone else is responsible to "do" us or make us feel good. Most women were raised to think that the man is going to make it right—and if he doesn't, we know whom to blame. Somehow, we think, he'll read our mind (magical powers that come with *true* love) and, presto, give us exactly what we want. The truth is that *we often don't know what we want*. So here's a good chance to spend some time with yourself experimenting. If we want our man to luxuriate over us for an hour of teasing, touching, and wooing, let's do it to ourselves.

SELF-TOUCH TECHNIQUES FOR WOMEN

Begin your self-pleasuring ritual by sitting in front of a mirror, giving yourself a heart salutation, and gazing into your own eyes. Connect with the sound of your breath coming into the nose and going out of the mouth with a sigh, as if fogging up a mirror. Voice aloud your intention for your self-loving ritual, such as, "I empower my sensual self to emerge," or, "I celebrate my sassy, sexy self." Observe yourself undressing. If your mind wanders off onto random thoughts, discipline it back to the present moment. Move slowly and deliberately, as if conducting a sacred ceremony. Step into the tub; feel every sensation.

As you luxuriate in the suds, practice sensate focus on yourself (focusing on your bodily sensations only). You are now both giver and receiver. Notice the subtle difference. Treat each pore, hair, and body detail as an aspect of the divine. Perhaps you'll try your new salt scrub or rubber-ducky vibrator. Slide the soap over your smooth skin. Resting your back on your bath pillow, explore how wet sensations, such as a hair shampoo, feel on your body. When ready, step out of the tub and pat yourself dry.

In front of the mirror, view your curves, your voluptuousness. Undulate to the music; dress up if you'd like. Touch your breasts. Play with your nipples with oiled fingers. Lubricate your vulva and tease your clitoris while watching yourself in the mirror. Note how eroticism softens your face. Massage the inner and outer vulval lips between your thumb and fingers. Slide a finger inside and rub the rough, spongy G-spot located about an inch inside, on the top surface of the vagina.

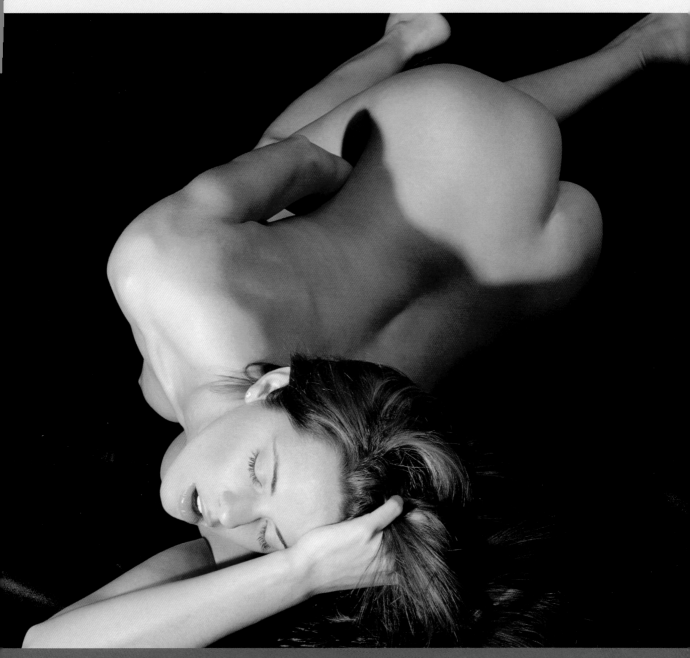

"At first I thought an hour of self-pleasuring would seem like forever, but it went so quickly. I had never looked in the mirror while I touched my genitals before. I liked what I saw. My lover is lucky to have such a brave, sexy lady."

—Tara, 39

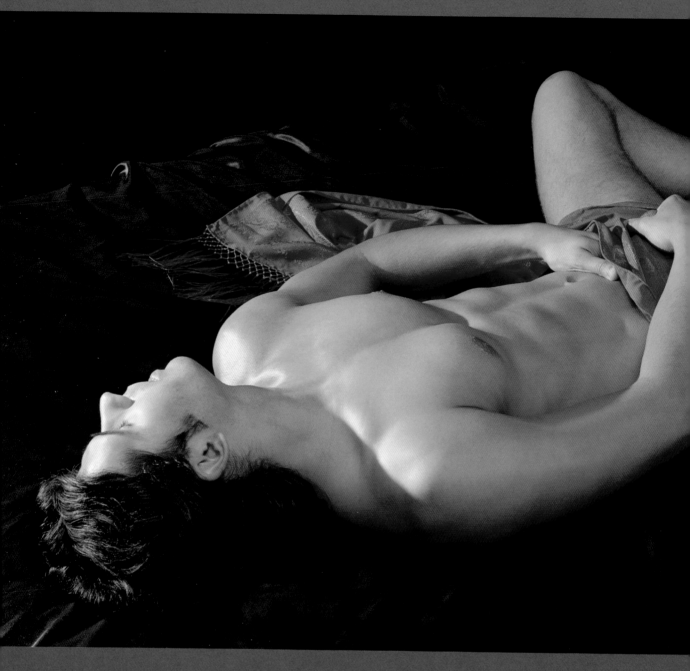

"*I remember a time when I carried one goal with my mastur-bation—to ejaculate. Old habits don't satisfy me anymore. Now I witness waves of pleasure, hear my heart race, and feel sensations that I compare to deep shocks followed by a thump-ing softness. My needs have changed.*"
—Shawn, 35

In self-pleasuring, a man can resensitize the penis and arouse himself with slower and lighter strokes, thereby more closely simulating the sensations of partner intercourse. Learning slower masturbation techniques will help prepare you to be a better lover.

Expand the edges of your experience. Witness in yourself the many faces of womanhood. Touch yourself as the virgin and innocent maiden. Grind your hips to unleash your lascivious self, the inner woman who knows how to lap up her pleasure shamelessly. See reflected in the mirror an erotic, passionate woman, creative and confident, who is claiming her sexuality.

Touch yourself however it pleases you. If orgasm happens, fine, but coming to orgasm is not the goal; rather, breathing into the pleasure of each moment is the intent. Close the ritual by sitting reverently in front of the mirror and honoring your erotic journey with a heart salutation. Call your partner and let him or her know you have completed your self-touching ritual. You may wish to share something about your experience or simply give thanks for the support.

MAN'S EROTIC SELF-MASSAGE RITUAL

As a man, you've been taught it's all about her. It's so important to please her that you forget to enjoy your own body or tune in to your own sensations. The responsibility you feel for "doing her" interferes with your ability to focus on your own body and learn the nuances of your arousal.

As men you've also been taught not to feel your feelings. The emotional body is off limits if you are to stay in control and be manly. Yet, to connect with a woman, you need to confidently negotiate the sensual, emotional body. Your old ways (quick and fast) of masturbating often work against your being able to connect with and fulfill your partner sexually. You can learn how to masturbate in ways that prepare you to be a better lover.

Through your solo-sex practice you can prepare yourself for prolonged, creative lovemaking with a partner that is richly sensual and free from performance anxiety. Conscious self-pleasuring strengthens your erections and orgasms and brings focus and potency to your loving. Improve your focus, attitude, and techniques of self-loving, and you'll have better sex with your partner.

SELF-TOUCH PREPARATION FOR MEN

For your solo-sex ritual, commit to spending an hour and choose an untraditional place—consider a private place, perhaps even one in nature if it's private!—or some other powerful place for you. If you usually masturbate in the shower, change the routine. Anchor yourself in deep, slow breathing. Visualize your inhale and exhale. Some men liken this expansion and contraction of the breath to the movements of lovemaking. Undress slowly and sensually.

SELF-TOUCH TECHNIQUES FOR MEN

Begin touching your whole body, unhurriedly, employing the sensate-focus techniques of focusing your attention on only where you are touching. Rub your chest, shoulders, and arms with lotion. If you generally lie down, try standing, or leaning against a wall (or tree, if you're outside). Look at yourself in the mirror. Move your hips, change your angle, and honor your unique male body and precious genitals.

Use oil or lotion on your penis, scrotum, perineum, and anus. Try lighter and slower strokes and take the time to feel each stroke. Touch the whole penis, including the shaft and the base. A reflexive organ like the hands and feet, the penis has different zones that relate to various internal organs. Change your grip, change hands. Massage other parts of your body while you stroke your genitals.

Be aware of how much pleasure you give yourself and your partner with this *wand of light*, a Tantric sex term for the penis. You are stroking a "wand" that creates new life and new souls.

Ejaculation is not the goal. Tune in to all your sensations and practice bringing yourself up and down in your arousal cycle. You're introducing your penis to new strokes, rhythms, and pressure. You may ejaculate (lasting a few seconds) or you may choose to remain in a prolonged orgasmic realm. You have a choice. Once you lose the single-minded need to always end in ejaculation, you begin a multifaceted journey into *high sex*, a Tantric term for accessing whole-body orgasms and multiorgasmic potential. Partner lovemaking becomes about the journey—not the destination. The man's prolonged attention is the key to transforming the ordinary sex into a spiritual union. Use the full hour, and end with an appreciative heart salutation.

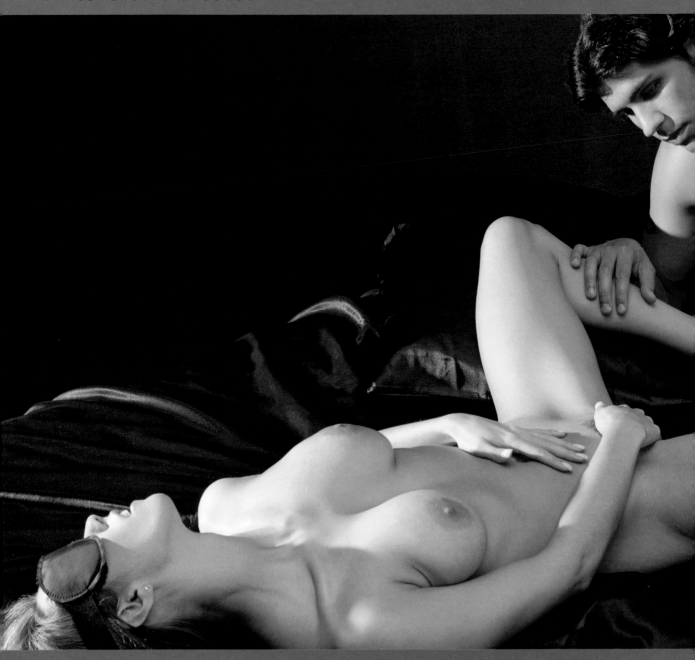

"*I was amazed how close I felt to my lover after I opened myself in this vulnerable way. I thought, 'If I can do this with him watching, I can tell him what feels good and what doesn't in partner sex.' This exercise helped me become more confident, which has really helped my sex life.*"

—*Laura, 29*

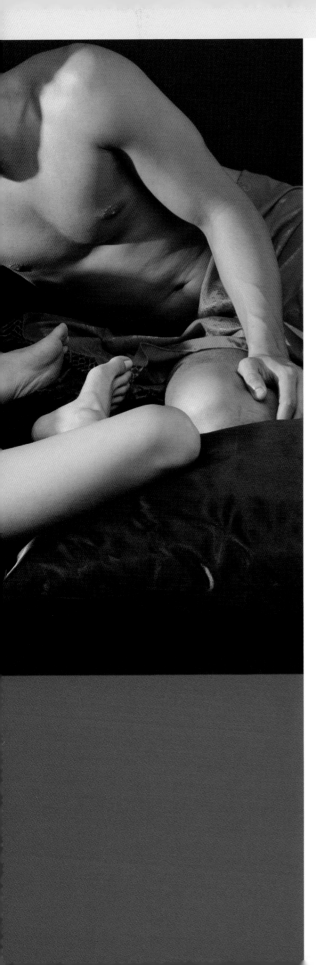

WOMAN SELF-PLEASURING FOR A MAN

One of the surest ways to quickly uncover layers of shame and liberate your innate creative sensuality is to pleasure yourself for your beloved. Sharing masturbation not only is instructive for your partner but empowers your sexuality in unfathomed ways. By witnessing each other in this most normal sex act, you drop the veil of secrecy and empower the root of eroticism—self-love.

PREPARATION FOR SHARING YOUR SELF-PLEASURING

As in the solo-pleasuring exercise, prepare your sacred space with all your silks, feathers, lotions, and oils. Invite your lover to get comfortable in some place in the room from which you wish him to observe. He remains nonverbal and nontouching in this exercise, though he may naturally breathe and sound with you. Position him where he can see your genital stroking. Allow thirty to sixty minutes for this exercise, and set the timer.

Begin by gazing into each other's eyes, synchronizing your breathing, and share your intention, "I intend to touch myself with appreciation." The witness may intend, "I intend to witness in gratitude your self-loving." Bow in a heart salutation. You may prefer wearing a blindfold. Either way, take the few minutes to close your eyes and come into your own breathing and body.

When you are ready, begin your self-caring ritual. Slowly undress (perhaps in front of the mirror), feeling the fabric swish against your skin. You are focusing on your sensations now, so when you remember you are being watched, gently bring your mind back to your body. Remember your solo-pleasuring experience. Share your authentic self, move to the music, smell the lotions, taste them on your skin. *Lavish yourself without feeling the need to please anyone else.* This time is for you. Take as long as you want doing luscious, wonderful things to yourself.

There is nothing sexier than a woman taking her pleasure. Be noisy with your breath, moan, groan, and squirm for your delight. When you're tired of doing one thing, invent another. Feather your feet, brush your hair, suck your fingers, and put warm oil on your nipples.

Warm up your pubic area with loving strokes. Massage your pubic mound, vulva, clitoris, and perineum. Use a generous amount of lotion, since the clitoris does not self-lubricate. Use your fingers, a vibrator, or a sex toy to penetrate your vagina if you feel like it. Relinquish the need for an outcome (such as getting wet or having an orgasm). Practice trusting, believing, and following your own desires, your own timing, and your own rhythm.

When the time is up, you may want to wash your hands and put on a robe and sit before your beloved. Take a few moments to tell him what the experience was like for you. He may respond with what it was like to witness you. This is not a time to suggest technique or to criticize but a time to report your own experience. End with a heart salutation and a hug.

MAN SELF-PLEASURING FOR A WOMAN

Women, like men, also appreciate seeing their lover fully exposed—both physically and emotionally. Practicing self-touch in front of your partner not only will enable you to become more comfortable with yourself but also will allow her to witness your vulnerability as a man, permitting her to feel an intimacy with you that she previously might not have felt.

PREPARATION FOR SHARING YOUR SELF-PLEASURING

Prepare your space, lubricant, lotions, and oils for your full-body conscious self-loving session with your lover as witness. Invite her to position herself comfortably where she can see you but not interfere with your movements (ideally not touching you). Set the timer for thirty to sixty minutes. Begin together by gazing, ocean breathing and speaking intentions, then bow in a heart salutation. She becomes the nonverbal, unobtrusive observer of your exploration.

"When this activity was first suggested by a sex coach I heard on the radio, I thought I would die. How could I expose myself? And I was afraid to 'bore' someone with my lackluster routine. However, I was amazed at myself before the hour was up. I was motivated to new levels of play simply by being observed attentively and quietly by my partner. I felt validated and normal, like I had nothing to hide."

—Carol, 35

Your woman will learn more about how to stroke you when you self-pleasure for her.

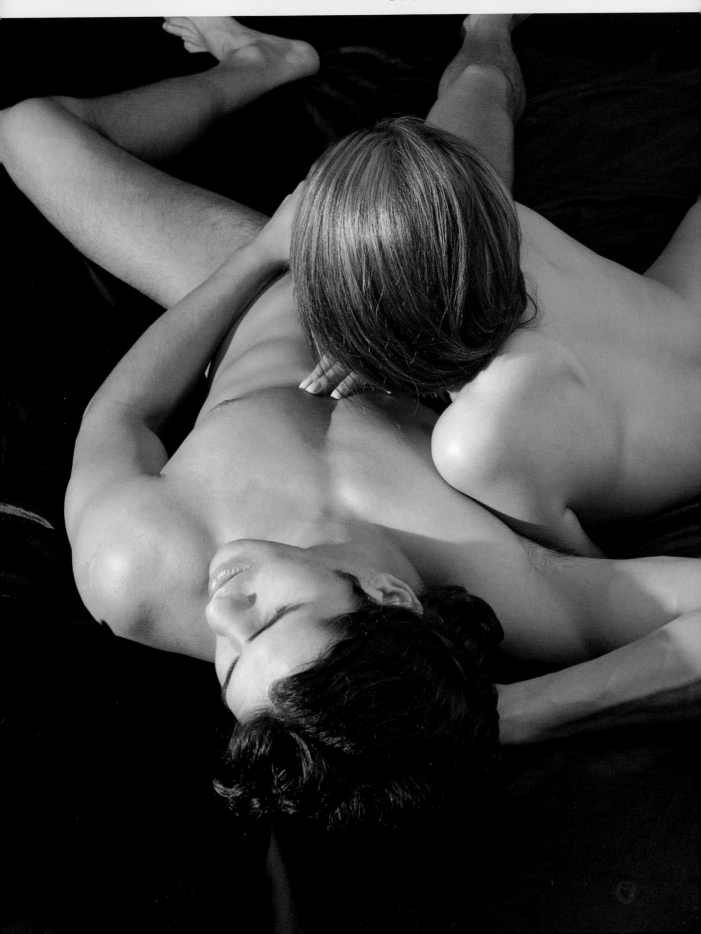

Breathe deeply with your eyes closed until you feel a connection to your intention, such as "to feel each sensation." Take your time. Massage your muscles with lotion, and feel your strength to protect, care, and provide for your loved ones and community. Massage your thighs and feel the power of your mobility. Touch your whole body. Wake up all the masculine aspects of yourself, the curious boy, the ardent lover, the foolish man, the wise and clever magician. Be awed by your versatility and depth.

Massage your genitals with the varied strokes you explored in your solo-loving practice. Allow your pleasure to flow with your breath and sound. Tease yourself. She will be fascinated. But you are not doing this for her. You are acknowledging yourself as a powerful, creative being capable of giving and receiving deep pleasure. Choose whether or not you will ejaculate, being fully aware that each time you have a choice. When you choose to delay ejaculation, you enlarge your capacity to hold larger amounts of erotic energy before spilling out.

When the time is up, wash your hands, put on a robe and sit before your beloved. Share with her your experience of being observed, and she will respond with her experience of observing. End with a heart salutation, a hug, or relaxation bonding.

WHEN A MAN CHOOSES TO BUILD EROTIC ENERGY without release, he signals to a woman that he is still attentive. In the East, ejaculation is described as "going," not "coming." After reaching climax, a man is literally depleted and needs a rest; his vitality and drive are diminished. Delaying ejaculation is a powerful tool to prolong the special relationship between lovers during sex.

"When my lover watched me self-pleasure, I felt very connected to my sexuality. I could focus on myself, because I wasn't trying to initiate or respond to her. It was very liberating, as well as extremely hot, to have her witness me in this state. I felt a deep appreciation for both her and myself."

—Tony, 46

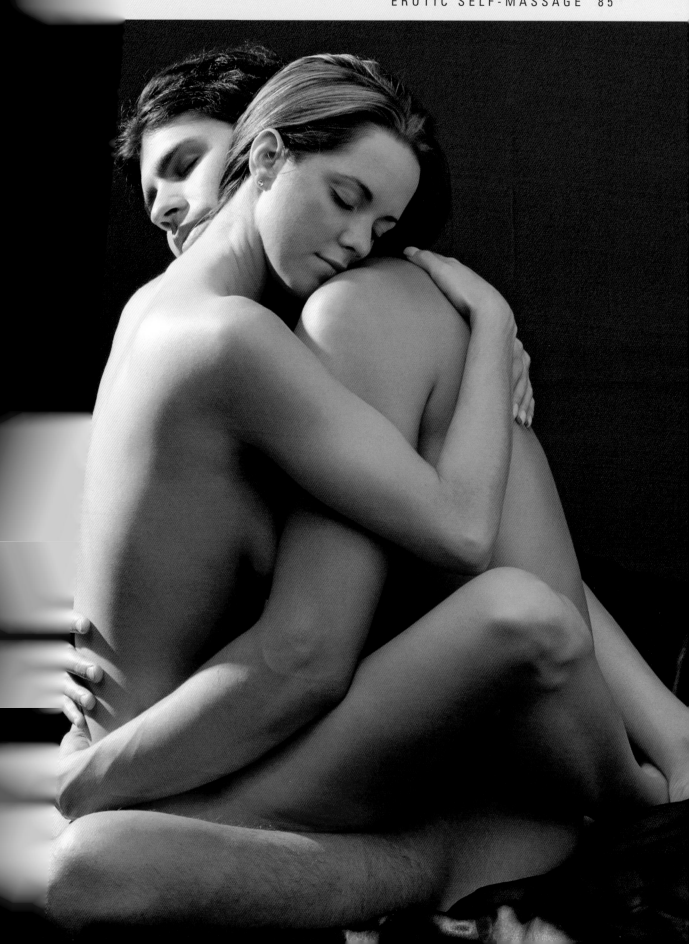

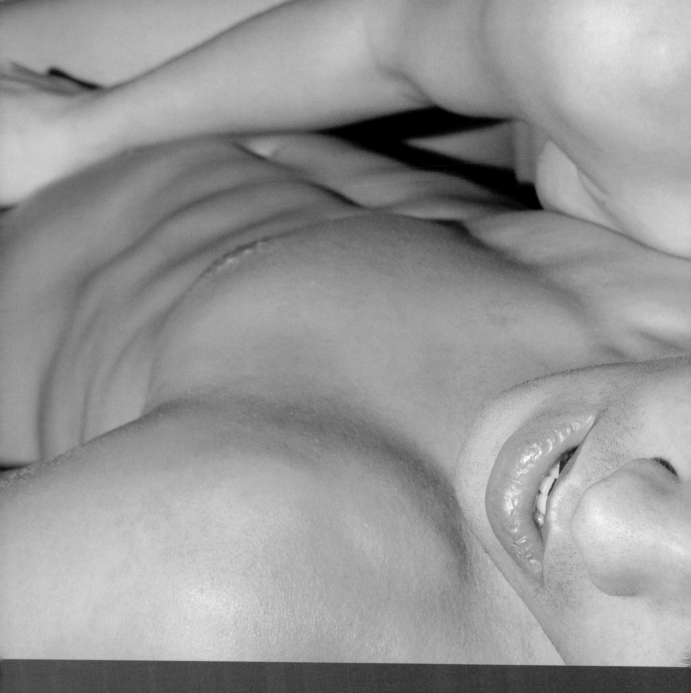

chapter
SIX

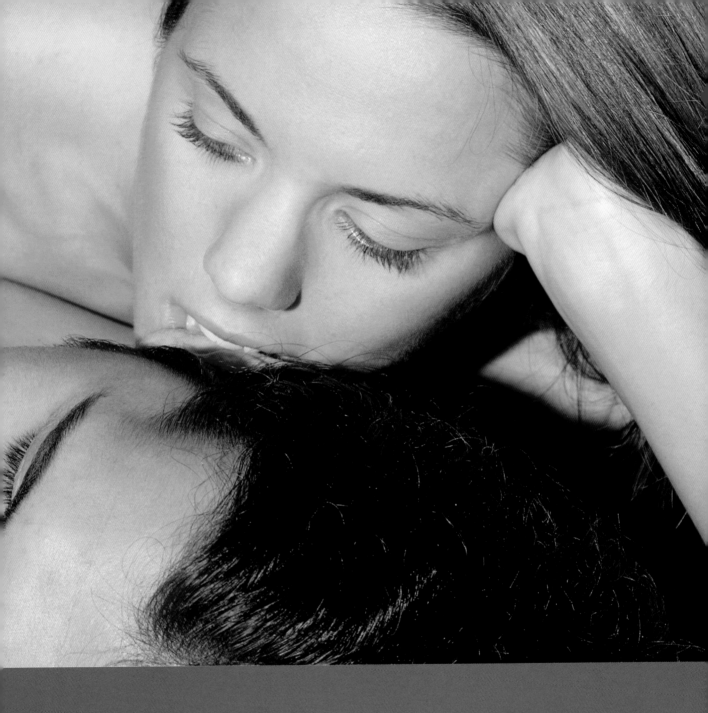

EROTIC GENITAL MASSAGE

GENITAL MASSAGE
TECHNIQUES FOR HER

The first time my partner offered me a genital massage, just to honor me as a divine being, I was nervous. I'd been touched there before only to be "prepped" for intercourse, and here was a sincere offer of massage for its own end. I was self-conscious, even embarrassed, to think of his touching my genitals without my giving back. I was afraid I would not perform for him by getting wet or having an orgasm. I wanted to say no.

I'm glad I got over that hurdle. True, it took me many times before I relaxed into the beauty of receiving fully, but the journey has been worth the risks. It's helpful for men to remind their women that this gesture is to be enjoyed as an end in itself. Your gift of a genital massage is not a stepping-stone to intercourse but a romantic and sensual bequest in its own right.

HEART AND GENITAL HOLD

After at least thirty minutes of nongenital body caressing or massage, ask her if you may honor her with a twenty-minute genital massage. By now she knows you are a man of your word. With her permission (and with short, smooth fingernails and clean hands), seat her comfortably in pillows, set the timer, place your hand over her heart and genitals, gaze and breathe. Express your intention, "I wish to nurture your holy well," or "I will allow you to feel your feelings." Ask her for her intention (expressed in positive language).

INDIRECT CLITORAL STIMULATION

Maintaining eye contact and keeping a hand on her pubic mound lightly touch with the other hand her chest, abdomen, and thighs with soft, long connecting strokes. Tell her she is safe with you; there's nothing she has to do except breathe, follow the touch, and be. Place one hand on her heart, the other palm over her vulva, and round your fingertips over the pubic bone. This is "heaven's back door" to the vagina's internal G-spot. Rotate your entire arm and wrist back and forth about an inch, firmly wrapping around the pubic bone. Check with her. She may feel a tingling internally. Hold and vibrate.

Ask her to lie supine, place pillows under her knees, and sit or lie beside her. Pour warm massage oil over the hand that is resting on her genitals, letting it filter through to the vulva. Hand over hand, use upward strokes from the perineum, spreading the oil over the entire genital region. The main center of pleasure for

Road to Intimacy

Genital massage opens a woman to her very core, and she needs to be aware of how unexpressed anger can interfere with turn-on and, therefore, orgasm. Oftentimes, this anger is directed toward her closest partner. Both men and women need to recognize and take responsibility for their anger and know that anger, no matter how justified, will not bring an ounce of happiness.

In life (and erotic massage) women often expect their male partners to be mind readers. We think that , "If he loves me, he'll know just what I want and magically give me everything without me asking." In this guessing game, both parties lose. Women withhold what they want, then blame men for not giving it to them. By choosing joy over anger, a woman can teach a man how to touch and gratify her. Most men want to gratify their partners and are capable of climbing mountains if they know what to do.

Communicate how you like your genitals to be touched and appreciate his efforts to pleasure you. Appreciation spawns intimacy.

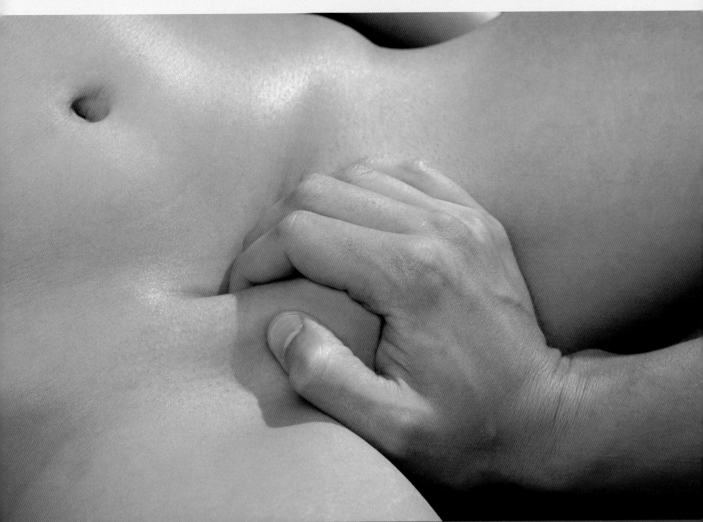

Opening "heaven's back door."

women is the clitoris, a tiny glans the size of a lentil with more than 8,000 nerve endings. Its only purpose is for pleasure, and since estrogen does not affect it, with stimulation it grows more sensitive as a woman matures. Most women need direct or indirect stimulation of the clitoris to orgasm.

Vulva Stroke

A. The vulva stroke stimulates the clitoris indirectly. Using your thumb and index finger, pinch a good amount of her outer lips (labia majora) and knead till it slips out of your grip. Continue from the clitoris to the perineum and back up the other side.

Give her love pats, with your flat fingers tapping the clitoris. Ask her about the pressure. Pinch the shaft of the clitoris from above, through the hood, and shake lightly. With both hands, pull the outer lips outward, while simultaneously starting at the inner lips (labia minora), spreading them toward where the thigh meets the pelvis.

Vulva Valley Stroke

B. For the vulva valley stroke, place one hand on her abdomen, and with your other hand, place a finger on each side of the clitoris and dip into the valley that runs down each side of the vaginal opening. Ask her if she wants more or less pressure, or a faster or slower speed. Vary this stroke with rhythm, pressure, and vibration. Use your fingertips to circle the clitoris. Ask her if you are in the right place, or how you could move to make it better. Circle in the other direction, and make circles around the vaginal opening.

MORE DIRECT CLITORAL STIMULATION

Clitoral Hood Strokes

C. With the palm on the pubic mound, stroke the clitoris with your index finger while you massage her inner thighs with the other hand. Retract the hood, exposing the glans, and find out what pressure she likes. Slide the hood back and forth without touching the clitoris with your fingers. Remember to stroke for a few seconds, pause, then vary the stroke in some way. Many women like close but not direct stimulation on the clitoris. Ask your lover. Include stillness with deep breathing as a stroke.

Often when we get to the genitals, our sensate-focus practice flies out the window. We get so nervous we hold our breath. Touch for your pleasure; enjoy this juicy, pink, soft part of her. To keep your focus, come back to your breath, intention, and touch.

Teasing the Clitoris

D. Tease the clitoris through the hood with your finger. Make sure there is plenty of oil or lubricant, because, unlike the vagina, the clitoris makes none of its own. Try exhaling some hot breath right onto the magic button; try a cool stream of air. Try a vibrator held on top of your hand that's touching her clitoris. The vibrations through your fingers will feel marvelous.

The Healing Power of Massage

All of us, women and men, have had negative sexual experiences: Perhaps we weren't ready for penetration yet, or we wanted to cuddle instead of have intercourse, or we started down that road, changed our minds, but couldn't express our desires. Some of us have been touched inappropriately when we were powerless to do anything about it. Women may have difficult issues regarding abortions, miscarriages, or childbirth. Negative imprints such as these are often stored in the genitals—and the cumulative effect is pelvic numbness and fear of sex. Genital massage with the intention to heal liberates and frees past patterns that have blocked us from our sensual feelings. Intentional erotic massage increases our body's sensitivity. Each of us decides how much we will release of past disappointments and anger. The more you let go, the more passion fills the new space.

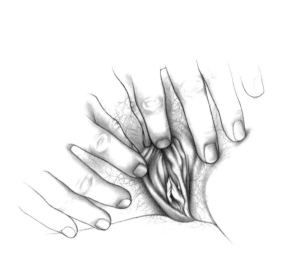

A. *Vulva stroke*

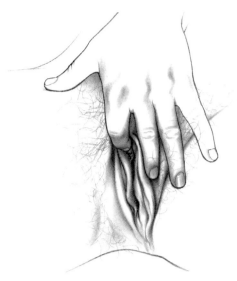

C. *Clitoral hood strokes*

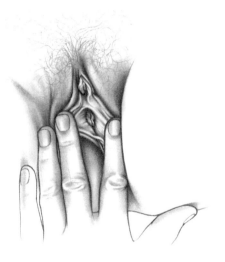

B. *Vulva valley stroke*

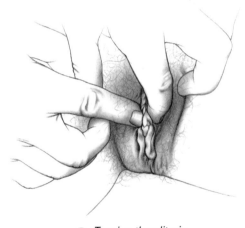

D. *Teasing the clitoris*

Talking to Her

Try being verbal with this massage. Tell her how beautiful her "flower" is. (Most women don't believe their genitals are beautiful.) If you notice her lips changing into a deeper pink or purple, tell her. If you see some wetness glisten from her vagina, remark how gorgeous it is. If her glans swell, tell her how bulbous her clitoris has become and how that makes you feel. You may also choose to stay nonverbal, but never tell her anything you don't truly feel.

Model deep surrender for her by sighing on your exhale. When she makes even a tentative sound, tell her how sexy her sighs and moans are to you.

Remember when she courageously self-pleasured for you? Mirror the same strokes she did on herself while solo loving. You could ask her to show you again how she did a certain stroke. She may or may not choose to maintain eye contact with you during this intimate encounter, though you may ask her to look into your eyes if you desire.

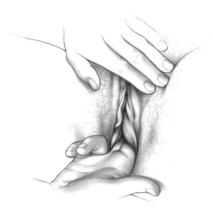

E. *Penetration*

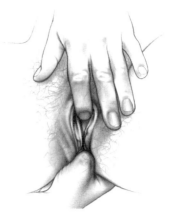

F. *G-spot or sacred spot massage*

VAGINAL MASSAGE

After spending at least five minutes stimulating the clitoris with plenty of lube, ask your lover, "May I touch you inside?" Or, "May I enter your temple gates?" Or, "May I visit your secret garden?" Look directly into her eyes and, using your own words, ask for permission in your most adoring voice. Staying on the outside of the vaginal canal is always a perfect option for either of you. If she does say no, it is often more about what's going on inside her than your technique. "No" is a precious gift; tell her "Thank you," and feel assured that in the future you can trust her "Yes."

Penetration

E. If she says yes, do not rush through the door. Linger seductively at the opening. Tease. Flirt. Picture her begging. Instead of friction, wait till you feel her sucking your finger into her essence. You may tell her, "Breathe me in." And if you don't feel a draw, wait. When ready (and with lots of lube), slowly penetrate her. Place one hand on her abdomen and slide one or two fingers all the way into the vagina, then hold still.

Use your sensate-focus skills, focusing your total attention on your bodily sensations. Notice the heat and moistness within this deep cave. With your whole hand, slide slowly in and out about an inch. How slowly can you move? Vibrate your hand lightly. Press in the four directions—upward, outward toward each leg, and downward—coming to the center and pausing a few seconds between each press.

G-Spot or Sacred Spot Massage

F. Pull your fingers back out to the second knuckle and curve them toward the pubic bone in a come-hither gesture, lightly stroking the top wall of the vagina. Feel for an area that is more spongy and wrinkly than the surrounding smooth tissue and about 1.5 inches inside. This sensitive area, about the size of a quarter, is connected internally to the clitoris. If the G-spot is touched before a woman is clitorally stimulated, it is unengorged and hard to find, and she feels nothing, or it is even painful (think of the head of your penis). At first a woman may feel the urge to urinate, but with a couple of slow breaths, that will pass.

Once you have found the sacred spot (with her help), make small circles with the flat pads of your fingertips. Pause. Change direction. Pause. Try the doorbell. Press up firmly toward the top of the pubic bone, hold five seconds, then release five seconds. Ask her about the pressure. Repeat several times. Make a windshield-wiper stroke in the same fashion.

Alternating Clitoral and G-Spot Stimulation

With one palm anchored on the pubic bone, use your fingers to manipulate the clitoris. Use your internal fingers or thumb of the other hand to massage the G-spot. Stimulate five to fifteen seconds on one spot, rest for a couple of breaths, then continue to stimulate the other spot. Resting your palm on the pubic bone helps her feel secure. Encourage your partner to feel her feelings and to breathe deeply.

CLOSING MASSAGE RITUAL FOR HER

A couple of minutes before the end of the massage, tell her, "I'm coming out from deep inside you now." Pause, then remove your internal hand *slowly* while the other hand rests on her lower abdomen. Rest your hot, moist hand over her genitals, and with the other one, massage around the heart, breasts, shoulders, and thighs, connecting the body to the genitals. End with a heart salutation, relaxation bonding, or mutual sharing if desired. As in all massages, with experience you may mutually decide to extend the time.

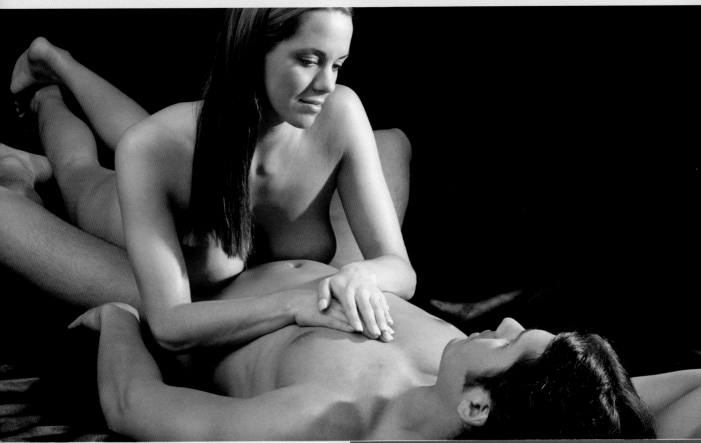

"*I never thought about asking for permission to enter my lover with a finger, and it felt pleasantly old-fashioned. It felt great being inside her after I received her blessing to be there. Asking permission no longer feels clinical to me, it feels deeply caring and intimate.*"

—*Stephen, 40*

Genital massage with the intention to heal liberates and frees us from past patterns that have blocked us from sensual feelings.

Keeping Time

As the active partner, you are the time-keeper. The giver must be aware of time and orchestrate a seamless massage progression from the opening ritual to closure. Don't get caught by the timer and be only halfway through the massage. Plan your time—in this case, for example, opening ritual five minutes, clitoral strokes five minutes, vaginal/clitoral strokes eight minutes, and closing ritual two minutes. Put your timer where you can see it.

GENITAL MASSAGE
FOR HIM

Bring your man deep into his body with thirty or more minutes of body caresses and/or massage, then ask him if you may massage his genitals. Clear permission here creates trust and safety. Tell him that for the next twenty minutes you want to massage his silky, pink parts for your pleasure. Remind him there's nothing he has to do but lie back, breathe deeply, and focus on his sensations.

THE GROUND RULES

Assure him that getting hard, or staying hard, or ejaculating is not expected—if it happens, that's okay, but it's fine if it doesn't. Men often report that they are never granted this permission, but when given, it is extremely freeing. Without the pressure to perform, a man is free to feel his own sensations and arousal, a necessary step in learning ejaculatory mastery.

Tell him that it is fun to play with a "soft-on" and medium-hard penis and you imagine it feels good to him, too. Tell him if he ejaculates in the first few minutes, you still get to touch his gorgeous parts for twenty minutes. *Commit to your own pleasure.* Tell him you will do only what feels good to you. Remind him he's not taking care of you now, he's receiving, which is often a difficult role for men.

COMPASSION FOR HIM

As a man ages, he requires more time and stimulation to get an erection, which is more tentative, and he needs to ejaculate less to maintain potency. The fact that a man might not respond to you "erection-wise" as in younger years doesn't mean he loves you less or is no longer attracted to you. Women need to have compassion for men whose sexuality is so exposed. Sometimes penises can become erect when nothing sexual is happening, or not get erect when they feel sexy and aroused.

HEART AND GENITAL HOLD

Set the timer. Position your breasts over his penis and place your hands over his heart. The man is strongest in root sexual energy, while the woman is strongest in the heart-love energy. In this position, you nurture and balance each other. Gaze and breathe together, basking in the flow of your complementary strengths. Speak your intention, such as, "I will nurture and heal your precious wand." His intention may be, "I open myself to feel each sensation."

GENITAL MASSAGE STROKES
FOR HIM

Begin by stroking his chest, abdomen, and thighs in long, smooth, connecting strokes. Vibrate his penis through your breasts by sighing aloud. Let your throat be soft and let the sound fall from your heart into his penis. Undulate between his legs. Marvel at the male playground before you.

In my sex-coaching practice, I'm surprised how often men tell me their women just want to "do it" quickly. It is good to hear that men also like to play, meander, and luxuriate in sensual touch. Here's your chance to honor him. Change position and sit between his legs, facing him, with his thighs over your thighs, or sit to his side if you prefer.

Pour some warm oil on top of your fingers covering his genitals and let it filter through. Alternating hands, stroke and spread the oil over the entire region. Tickle the pubic hair, stroke his balls, and take a generous pinch of scrotum skin, pulling up on it and kneading it between your thumb and fingers. Shake it. Work all around the scrotum and perineum, stretching and pulling.

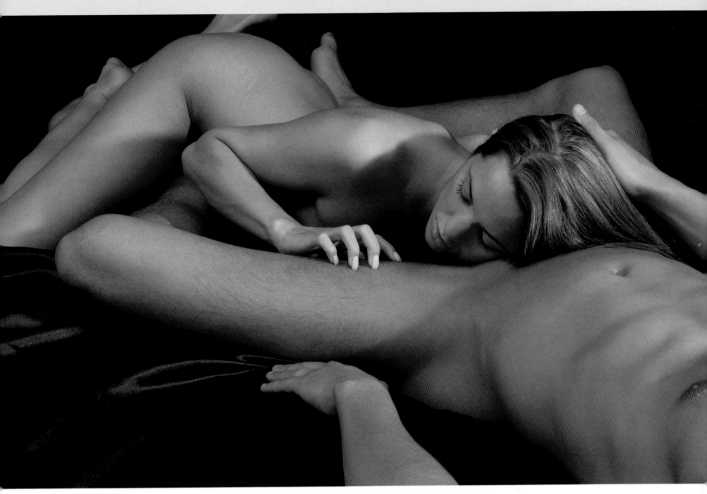

Tell you partner to simply observe his arousal without trying to withhold or heighten it during a genital massage. Remind him to relax, breathe deeply, and focus on his sensations.

Perineum Stroke

A. With one hand on his penis, make a fist with the other hand and dig deep into the "hidden penis," also known as the *perineum*. Rotate and vibrate your fist. Lean into it with your whole body. Check with him for more or less pressure. This area loves touch and is usually ignored. You may wish to review perineum massage from chapter 3, under "Back Body Massage." Open your fist and place the palm over the perineum with thumb and finger encircling the scrotum. Press and massage firmly from this angle.

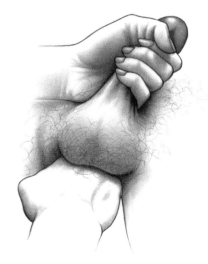

A. *Perineum stroke*

Scrotum Stretch

B. For the scrotum stretch, encircle one hand around the balls, with your fingers touching on the underside; and with the other hand on the shaft of the penis, pull gently in the opposite direction. While stretching in opposition, try stroking his balls with your fingers on his scrotum. Remind him to keep his thighs, butt, and abdomen soft.

Around-the-Clock Stroke

C. In what I call the around-the-clock stroke, you massage the scrotum with one hand while you take the penis in the other and rotate it in a circle, as if it were a hand of a clock. Squeeze playfully from base to tip at every hour. Pay special attention and more time at the six-o'clock "good news" position and the twelve-o'clock "healing" position, where your stroking hand can continue up to the heart.

Hold the base of the penis while you stroke the sensitive area beneath the head on the underside of the penis, the frenulum. Pulling the skin taunt at the base increases the sensitivity at the head.

Corkscrew Stroke

D. You can do a corkscrew stroke by twisting the penis shaft and head as you slide your hand up and down. Remember to pause occasionally to allow the sensations to subside. As when stroking your own clitoris, intersperse pauses. Vary your pressure and speed and check in with him.

Massage the shaft, not just the head, of the penis. With one hand covering the penis, massage the inner thighs in a U stroke (the stroke can also extend all the way to the heart) with your other hand. Use a vibrator against the hand holding the penis. If he tenses his thighs, touch them and ask him to make them soft. Being relaxed combined with deep and even breathing helps him contain more sexual energy. Press under the scrotum to help bring him down from high levels of arousal.

VALIDATE HIM

Most men think their penises are too small. The average penis when erect is five and a half to six inches (porn movie stars don't count!). Some men have big nonerect penises that only slightly enlarge with stimulation; other men have smaller nonerect penises and grow substantially with arousal. Either way, make a point of sincerely telling him how this precious part of him pleases you.

Describe how beautiful the mushroom head is shaped, or the veins on the shaft, or how it turns deep

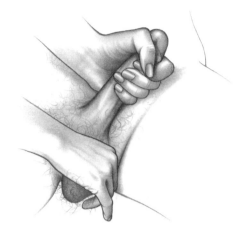

B. *Scrotum stretch*

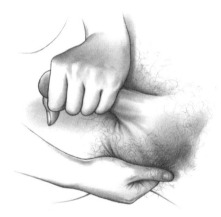

C. *Around-the-clock stroke*

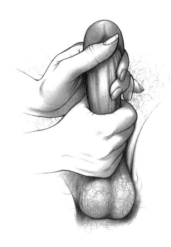

D. *Corkscrew stroke*

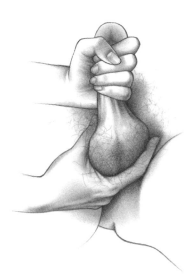

E. Press and massage the perineum while you stroke the penis.

Tell your lover how beautiful you find all parts of his body.

purple with arousal, and how perfect its size is for you. Remark how big his penis looks from your view (they judge it from only one angle—and not the best one!). Tell him how it feels to have your hand around his hardness and how much pleasure you derive from him.

Remember the strokes you watched him perform on himself when he self-pleasured for you? If so, duplicate these strokes as you play with him. Women are often too tentative with touch because they relate it to the sensitivity of the clitoris. Remember the pressure he used on his own balls and mimic it. (See figure E.) If in doubt, ask him if he wants more or less pressure.

If it feels like work, you may be performing for him or trying to make him come. Back off. Stop, breathe, find your center, and think of your intention. It has nothing to do with outcome, and everything to do with the journey. This is different from the usual. Allow yourself the freedom. If he happens to ejaculate, encourage him to enjoy the explosion, and invite him to stay with his sensations. Wipe him off with a warm, wet towel and continue your massage, avoiding the tip of the penis, which can be supersensitive after orgasm.

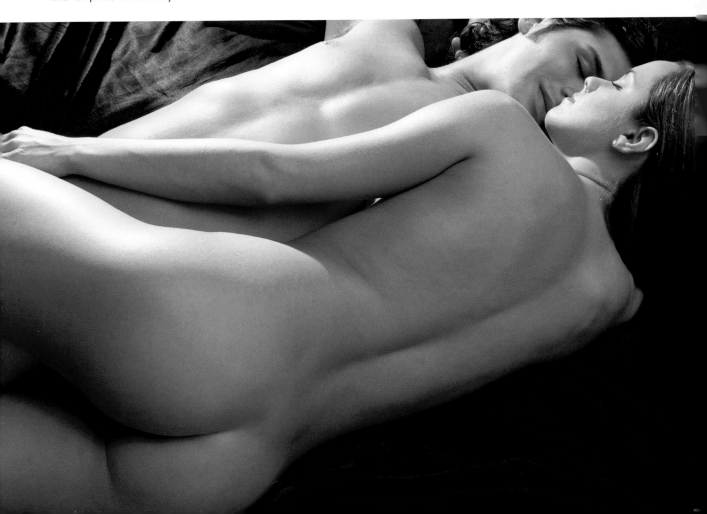

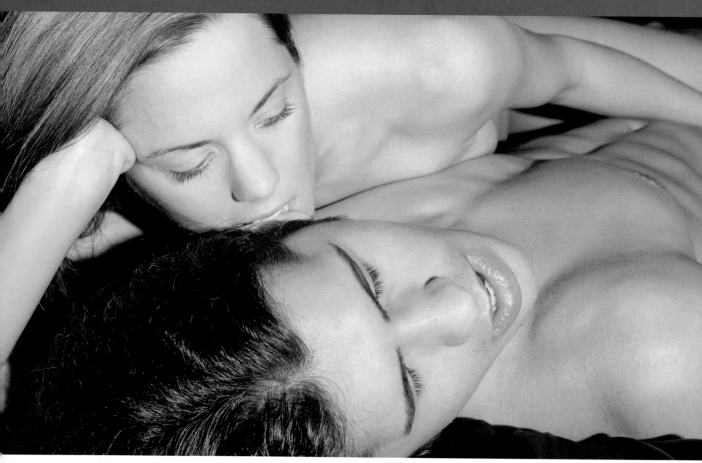

Prolong and heighten your partner's arousal with light and varied strokes.

"The key for me was when she said I didn't have to get hard and I didn't have to do anything. That was so different. I realized how much pressure I put on myself all the time. When she massaged me, I felt relaxed and excited at the same time. Taking turns has helped me fully feel all my sensations."

—Richard, 32

CLOSING MASSAGE RITUAL FOR HIM

A couple of minutes before the end of the massage, slow your strokes and cover his genitals with one hand while you massage his chest, shoulders, and heart with the other hand. It feels unusual to massage a man's genitals without the purpose of making him ejaculate. Your self-worth may come into question. His self-worth may come into question. You are learning to contain more erotic energy in a prolonged orgasmic realm.

Containment of sexual energy is the juice that lubricates flirting, attention, desire, and seduction in a relationship. Containing arousal is not often practiced in relationships. Boredom and routine come from thinking every sexy touch needs to end in orgasm. With

your hand, cover the underside of his penis and, with the other hand covering his heart, breathe in the wonder of the moment together. Share with him how powerful his aliveness feels to you. End in a heart salutation, bonding, or mutual verbal sharing.

PROLONGING AROUSAL TECHNIQUES FOR **HIM**

Most couples want to prolong and heighten the special rapport that comes from erotic massage and lovemaking. Men seek ways to prolong their arousal so they can be more available to support women's pleasure. The tools for prolonging sexual energy, many of which the men have already practiced in this book, are simple. *Developing a slow, even and deep breath is fundamental to extending ecstasy. Without it you cannot focus on your sensations and learn how to go up and down in your arousal cycle.*

By relaxing your big muscles, such as thighs, buttocks, and abdomen, you can hold more erotic energy; tensing muscles makes you need to ejaculate. *Being relaxed while excited* seems foreign to us in the West, though Tantra teaches this technique as a means to cultivate and circulate erotic energy from the fiery root (genitals) throughout the entire body. Learn to recognize tension in your body and release it routinely to last longer.

Practicing conscious masturbation, as covered in chapter 5, makes the penis more sensitive to lighter and more varied strokes. This sensitivity encourages you to spend more time and involve the whole body to prolong arousal. If a man takes only a few minutes to masturbate and remains fixed on one type of hard, fast stroke for orgasm, and he assimilates this pattern to climax during intercourse, his partner will not feel satisfied. *Practice prolonging arousal in your solo loving.*

The PC (pubococcygeus) muscle is the pelvic-floor muscle that you tighten to stop the flow of urine. If exercised daily, it strengthens your erections, makes them last longer, and makes your orgasms stronger. *Pulse the PC muscle* every day and eventually hold for longer, sustained intervals. Similarly for women, the Kegel exercises strengthen the vagina, increase sensations for her and her partner, and make her orgasms more powerful. Much of Tantra, ancient sacred sexuality teachings, instructs how to use a strong PC muscle in conscious combination with breathing and movement to achieve prolonged ecstasy. Fortunately, many books on Tantra and becoming multiorgasmic are available today.

Once you have spent several weeks getting your PC muscle in shape, begin adding PC contractions to your self-pleasuring sessions. Ride the waves of your arousal with attention to your sensations, familiarizing yourself with your arousal process. At the peak of a wave, contract your PC muscle and firmly hold it. This will help bring you down.

The squeeze technique works similarly to contracting the PC muscle to avert ejaculation. Press your thumb and finger just under the rim of the glans or the head of the penis when you feel the urgency of climax approaching.

"*After two months of practicing, I was able to ejaculate only when I wanted: after my lover peaked several times and we gave each other the 'go for it' signal. We'd been making love for fifteen years, and this was such a gift to our intimacy.*"

—*Mark, 45*

The Start/Stop Technique for Men

In the start/stop technique, you stop stimulation before ejaculation seems inevitable. After a rest and subsiding of arousal, begin stroking again. Enjoy your practice sessions, including your mistakes. Extending the duration of your erection will be appreciated by your partner. Invite her to join you for some peaking exercises and decide on a nonverbal signal to stop stroking.

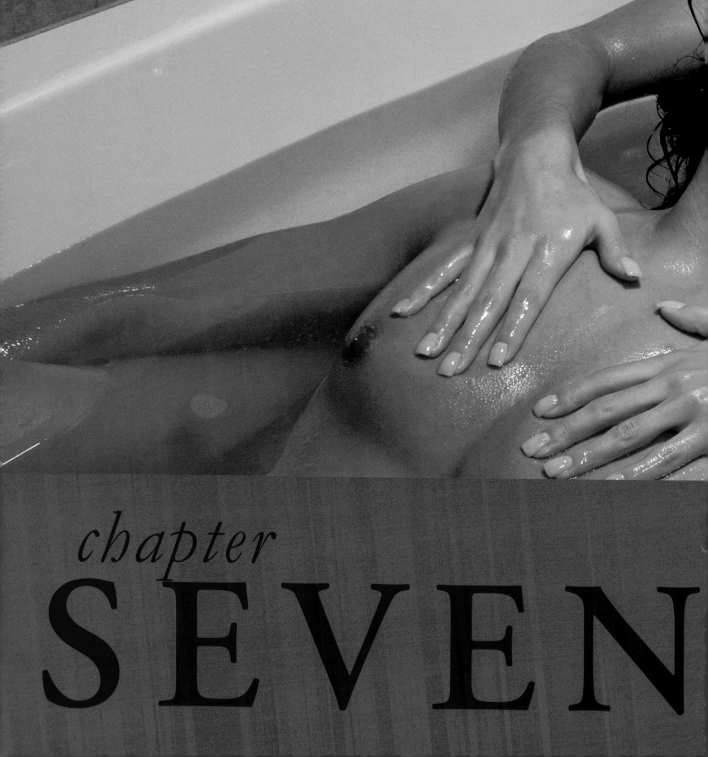

chapter

SEVEN

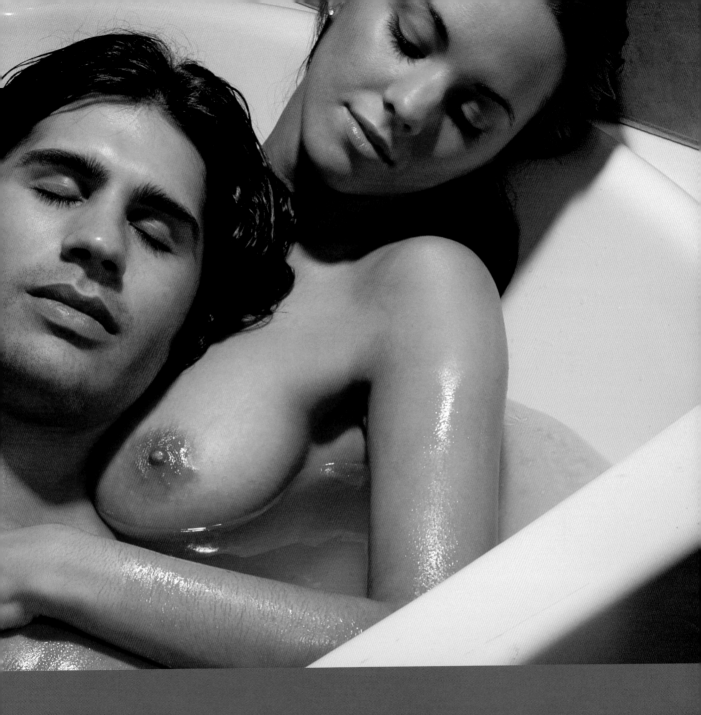

SENSUAL SHOWER
AND EROTIC BATH MASSAGE

THE SENSUAL
SHOWER

By now you have shared timeless and treasured moments exploring the body erotic with sensuous caresses and massages. Your enhanced skills of conscious breathing and touch can go anywhere with you—even to the shower. A warm, soapy shower will leave you feeling slippery clean and deeply nourished.

SOLO SENSUAL SHOWER

Often we hope a lover will please us for an extended time, yet we don't think of spending time satisfying ourselves. Luscious solo escapades are the foundation for partner exploration. Schedule an hour for a solo sensual shower. A shower is generally a quick and routine affair, so changing your speed and focus can be an adventure.

Prepare a warm bathroom in some special way and include aromatic soap to stimulate your sense of smell. Focus yourself by the opening ritual of breathing and intention. Step into the shower, feel the enclosed environment signal the opportunity to go inside yourself. Allow your troubles to trickle away and tune in to your sensations. You need only a little stream of water to keep the soap on your skin from drying.

Touch yourself from head to toe as you would a precious lover. Your skin isn't particular about who touches it, whether it's yourself or a lover; any sensation is welcome. Try applying a salt scrub; its rough texture makes your skin tingle but becomes smooth as stone when you wash it away. Feel the silkiness of soap on your genitals. What a great place to practice your conscious masturbation skills. Explore a new touch, lighter and slower than usual. Pump your PC muscle, which will tingle your genitals. If you're a man, enjoy prolonging your arousal by using the squeeze or stop/start technique. Expand your hard time by enjoying orgasmic sensations without the finality of ejaculation.

Touch your nipples and your vulva (or testicles if you're a man) and lightly stroke your anus. The anus is richly endowed with nerve endings, and after the clitoris and the penis, it is the body's most erotic zone. A soapy shower is a good place to get acquainted with this underappreciated (and overshamed) part of us. Lubrication, such as a soapy finger, is always a good idea for the delicate skin here. After touching the anus, wash your hand before touching other body parts. Often couples include anal touch (and sometimes penetration) as part of whole-body exploration.

End the sensual shower by patting dry and pampering yourself with lotions or other body-honoring rituals. Take extra time grooming the details of your body temple. Celebrate the sensual shower as an act of self-love. Taking responsibility for your own pleasure relieves your partner of always having to do it.

"Touching myself in the shower has both a calming and an erotic effect on me. As the warm water gushes down on me, I slowly trace my fingers around my nipples and my breasts, and then gently massage my clitoris. When I'm finished with it all, I am not only physically clean but emotionally refreshed and sexually satisfied."

—Julia, 34

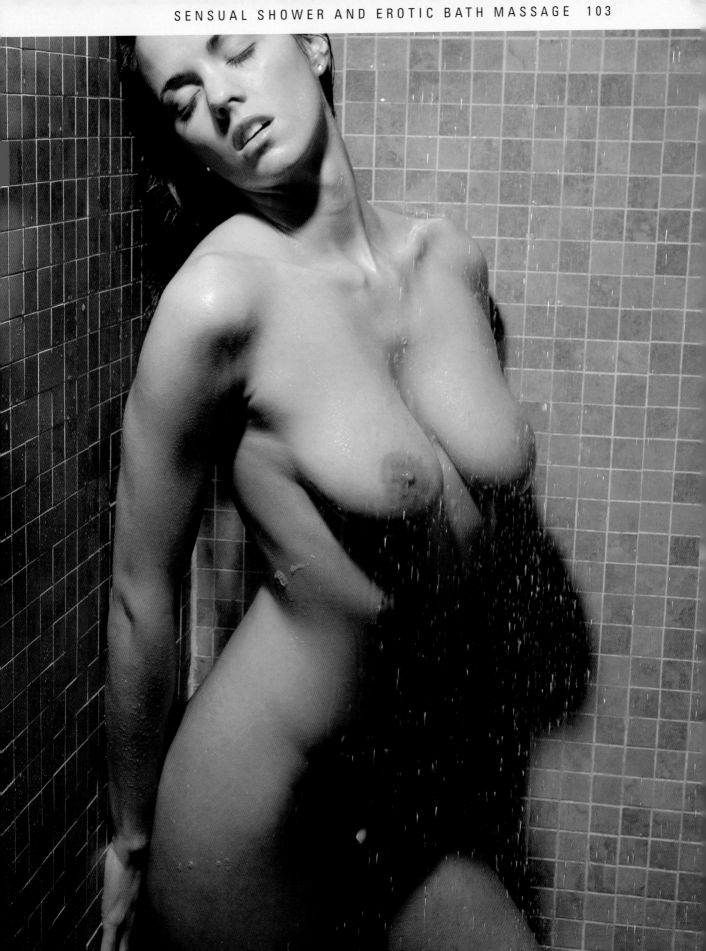

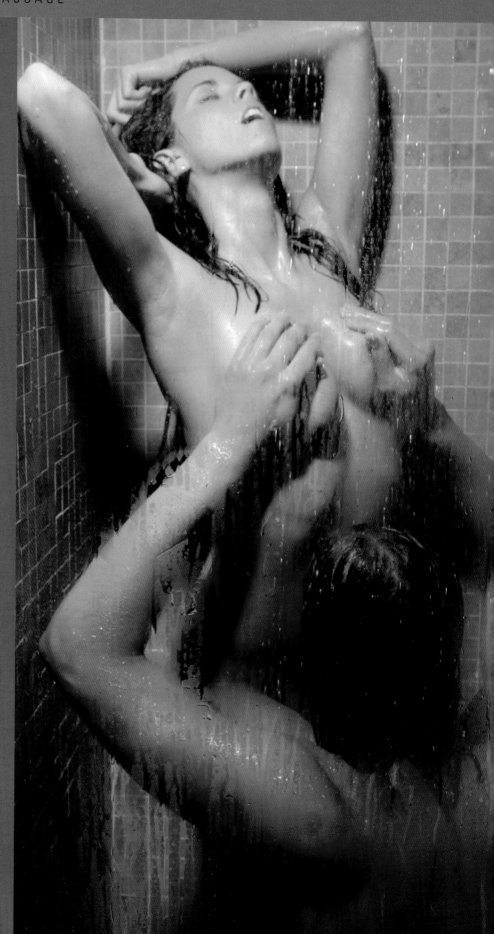

A woman's body pulls a man out of his head and into his body.

PARTNER SENSUAL SHOWER

Now you are ready to share a sensual shower with a partner. Decide who will first be the toucher (giver) and the touchee (receiver). The sensual shower is non-verbal. Set aside an hour and begin with a heart saluta-tion, gazing, breathing, and sharing intentions.

As the active partner, begin by lathering up your lover's back. Slip your soapy hand over her mounds and dips, noticing how different water feels from oil on dry skin. Rub your shoulders and your entire chest over her back and buttocks (she can brace against a wall with her hands). Try closing your eyes to heighten your sense of touch. Turn back-to-back with her and slip up and down her whole back body with your body. Be creative and move slowly so you can feel each movement and each breath.

Explore the front of her body like a child at play. If you should encounter an erect nipple (or penis, if the man is receiving), enjoy it casually and move on when you're ready. Linger at the genitals, but do not fixate on them. Honor the whole body with touch. Use all your body parts, including buttocks, hair, and tongue, to sense and taste your partner in the wet, steamy heat. Try a slow sensual shampoo.

Touching for your own pleasure is the key to sensu-ality. Often we try to guess what the other likes and "perform" it. Stay with what pleases you and you will be amazed at the results. If you are "performing" or worried about doing it right, you'll lose the joy of the moment. Do it for you. Remember, your touch is not about sexual stimulation-it's about sensual arousal.

In addition, don't forget to have wet fun with your partner! We open our hearts to joy and wonder by playing in the moment. Remember as children how our play followed no preconceived design; we just lost our-selves in the game. Sharing playful moments with your partner is essential for a strong emotional relationship. When you and your lover feel stretched and thinned by life's challenges, you'll have reserves to draw upon. Your shared pleasure is an investment that secures your relationship.

The sensual shower is enjoyed as an end in itself. It's not an appetizer for the main event-intercourse with the goal of orgasm. We are not striving for a desired outcome. If we were, we'd miss the experiences along the way. When we practice nonattachment to a speci-fied outcome, our striving ceases and we can enjoy the moment. About halfway through the sensual shower (thirty minutes), trade roles, and now the woman will become the giver.

Stop Performing and Start Enjoying

Touching for your own pleasure is the key to sensuality. Often we try to guess what the other likes and "perform" it. Stay with what pleases you and you will be amazed at the results.

ORAL MASSAGE IN THE SHOWER

Using the mouth in sensual massage creates sweet and juicy sensations and can develop deep intimacy. Oral massage can be practiced in the shower (or anywhere else, for that matter!). Here are some techniques to try during your partner shower or other activities.

Wet Oral Massage Techniques

Start with a relaxed mouth and soft lips; slightly protrude them without a huge pucker. Soft lips can feel more than tense, tight ones. Be gentle with kisses at the start; too much pressure numbs the mouth. Most women report that a good kisser starts light and gradually turns on the juice. Don't make the mistake of too much too fast.

Kneeling in front of him, barely brush your mouth over one of his hands. Lightly press a knuckle between your lips, then another. Kiss his hand lightly (no whiskers if you are a man). Open your mouth and trace the contours of his fingers with your tongue, especially between the fingers. Enjoy the silky sensations. Take a finger into your hot mouth, suck it in and out, going from light and slow to a more vigorous action. Roll your tongue around the finger for the joy of it.

Leisurely nibble your way up the forearm and kiss his shoulders. With a parted mouth, lick the water droplets off his collarbone. Feel his chest hair tease your lips. Suck his nipples. Never entirely release your suction-keep it minimal and move the nipple back and forth.

Delicately brush his earlobes with your lips, even pulling playfully. Flick your tongue over the contours and dips of his face. Drag a flat tongue over his neck and feel your hot breath behind it. Do what feels good to your tongue—lead with it. Nibble on his neck. Notice all the sensations. Feel how your tongue loves sensation. Lick some skin with a soft, flat tongue and then an erect tongue. Follow by blowing a stream of cool air.

Use your lips and tongue to massage your partner with awareness and joy. Discover how each square inch of your lover is a unique sensation to your mouth. Explore his eyelashes, earlobes, whiskers, nipples, penis, inner thighs, back of knees, toes, and fingers.

After the shower, take turns patting each other dry. Feel the heat of your bodies. Pamper each other with lotions and hair combing. End the ritual by finding your voice again and sharing one appreciation that each of you takes from the experience.

Use your lips and tongue to massage your partner with awareness and joy. Discover how each square inch of your lover brings a unique sensation to your mouth.

"I felt so cherished. I'll never forget our shower together; it felt so intimate and sacred. I went from making animal sounds and laughing to being spellbound by his gaze and caring touch."

—Ashley, 28

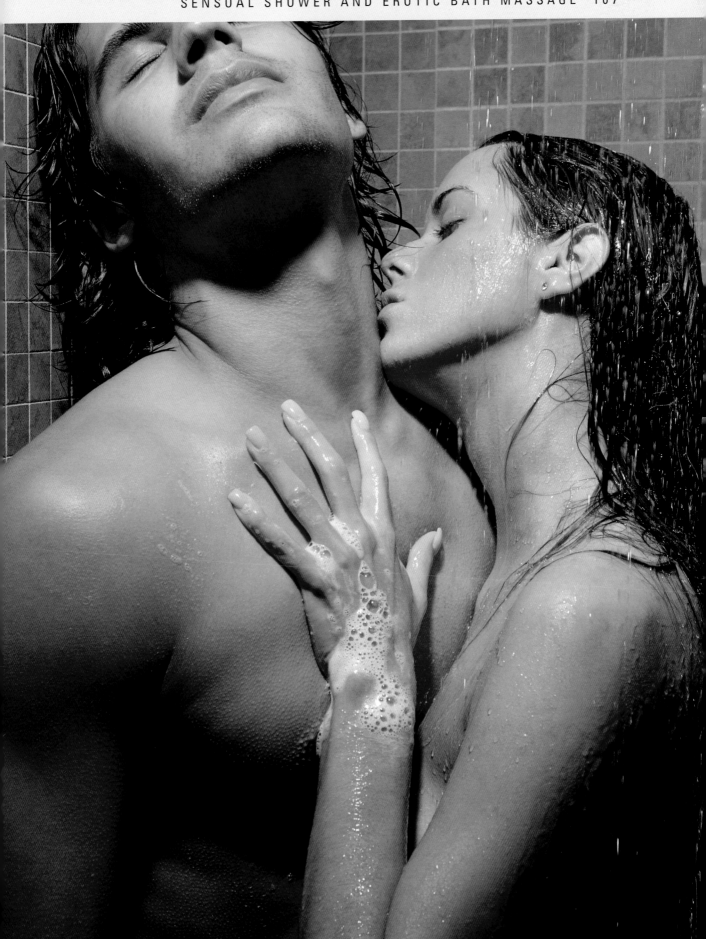

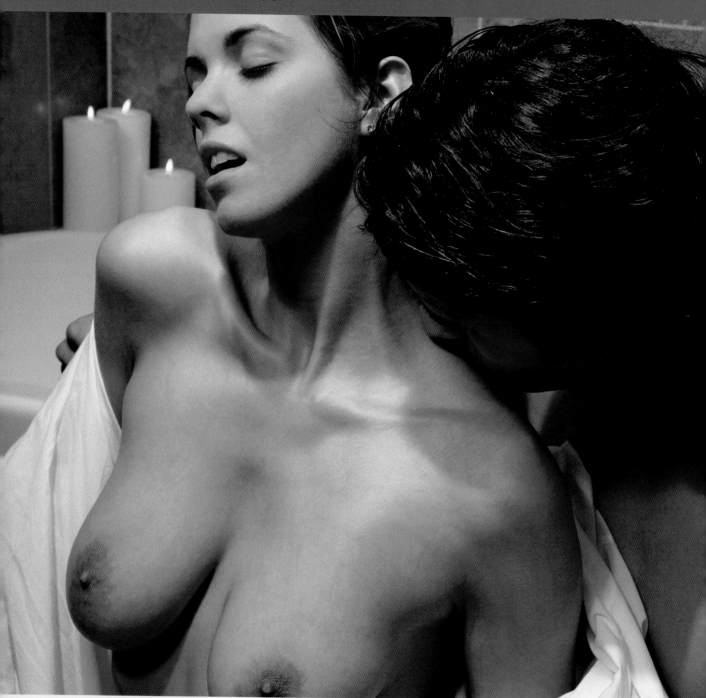

"Once a month my husband will surprise me—I never know when—by giving me what I now refer to as my 'sacred bath.' I'll come home from work and the bathroom will be filled with candles and flowers, the bathtub will be filled with bubbles, and he'll undress me and put me into the tub. He then massages my shoulders, my chest, my feet—wherever I want him to. Sometimes we make love afterward, sometimes not, but it is not about that. It's about his honoring me and my body, and I always feel like a queen during this loving and sensual act."

—Kara, 36

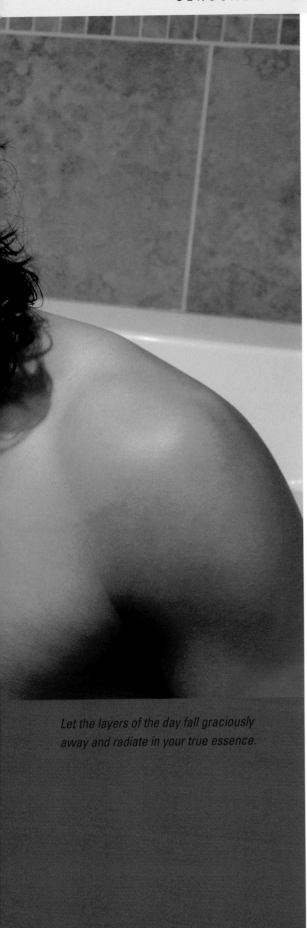

Let the layers of the day fall graciously away and radiate in your true essence.

BATH AND MASSAGE
CEREMONY

Honor your beloved with a timeless and euphoric bath and massage ceremony, one of the most fulfilling of all erotic encounters. This ancient ritual carries us back to the womb and resonates within us a primordial chord of deep pleasure and peace. Bathing a beloved is a humble and sacred act. Plan an entire evening for this reverent ritual, which will open both your heart and your lover's, healing, nourishing, and rejuvenating you.

PREPARE FOR YOUR PRINCESS

Invite your lover (in this case, the woman) to a night of sexual ecstasy. Give her a handwritten invitation or buy an erotic card. Enclose a feather. Dare to make the date for sometime in the future, and leave a couple of breathy voice messages or other hints of your passion in her path. Write or find a poem or prayer to express your reverence for her and buy her a gift (perhaps flowers) for the ceremony.

You, as prince of pleasure, prepare the bath and massage room with candles, incense, and her favorite music, and have wine or champagne on hand. Have a warm robe for your princess, two bath towels, a hand towel, a bath pillow, scented oils, a plastic pitcher, a large sponge, bath salts, and bubbles. You may want a pillow for yourself for kneeling or sitting beside the tub. Before she arrives, have the candles lit and the music playing. Pace yourself so you feel unhurried and centered. Dressed in a robe, greet her as you would a goddess.

CREATE SACRED SPACE TOGETHER

See the spark of the divine in her eyes. Kiss her hand and seat her on pillows in your sacred space. After a heart salutation, set the tone for your ceremony by purifying the space.

The following steps outline how to create sacred space.

1. **Clear away negative fears.**
   Clear away negative fears and doubts by offering something you're willing to let go. For example, "I let go of my worries from the day," or, "I rid myself of expectations for the ceremony," or, "I expel my fear that I'm not worthy of this honoring." Both of you share your doubts until they are all articulated. The mere mention of fears somewhat diminishes or disarms them. Allow the ritual to perform its magic.

2. **Offer positive affirmations.**
   Now you and your beloved offer positive affirmations to fill the space previously occupied by negativity. Take turns establishing positive energies with statements such as, "I call in compassion, truth, love," etc., or, "I invite in my playful self," or, "I call in nurturing energies." Name positive attributes to sanctify your space; conduct the ceremony in the style of a shaman.

3. **Share your intention.**
   Once you have cleared away mental obstacles and called in positive energy to shape the ritual, soul gaze into each other's eyes, breathing together for several minutes. Share your personal intention for this ancient ritual. Give her your gift and read her a poem.

Tell her you won't be talking much during the bath and massage ritual, so you both can rest calmly in the ecstasy of the moment, tuning the mind in to the sensual body. Invite your partner to surrender to her own pleasure, as you will be doing the same. Start filling the tub and keep a mental note (or timer) to turn off the water after the disrobing ritual.

DISROBE YOUR PRINCESS

In a seamless, slow-motion dance, take off her clothes. Let the layers of the outside world fall away as her true essence emerges. Draw out this seductive dance, flirting, and teasing. Slide the sleeve of a silky blouse up and down her arm and float it over her body.

Drape a warm robe around her shoulders and lead her to the bath chamber. Check the water temperature and help her step into the bubbly water. Position her deep in the tub (standard-sized bathtubs work just fine) with an inflatable bath pillow beneath her back and place a folded towel beneath her head. Wet the hand towel in the water and draw it up seductively between her legs to rest on her breasts and abdomen for added warmth. Hand her a glass of champagne.

BATHING HER

Once she's in the tub, make an energetic connection by gazing and breathing with your hands on her heart. Pick up the foot nearer you, nestle it in your arms, and wash, massage, and suck her toes. After five minutes on her foot, begin working up the leg, rubbing in fragrant salts, kissing her all over, and rinsing her off with a sponge or pitcher of water.

Reach for the other foot and serve your woman as if she were Queen of the Nile. Every few minutes, reimmerse the hand towel on her chest in hot water and pull it up over the genitals to rewarm her chest. Help her sip some champagne. Move to the arms. You are putting together everything you have practiced—arm and shoulder massage, a hand caress, and oral massage. Loll your tongue around the contours of her hand and fingers; feel the pleasurable sensations fill your mouth. Trust your own pleasure to guide you to the next stroke. Lick the inside elbow crease of her arm. Massage the tension of the day from her shoulders. Encourage her deep breathing by staying centered in your breathing.

Trust your own pleasure to guide you to the next stroke in a seamless, slow-motion dance.

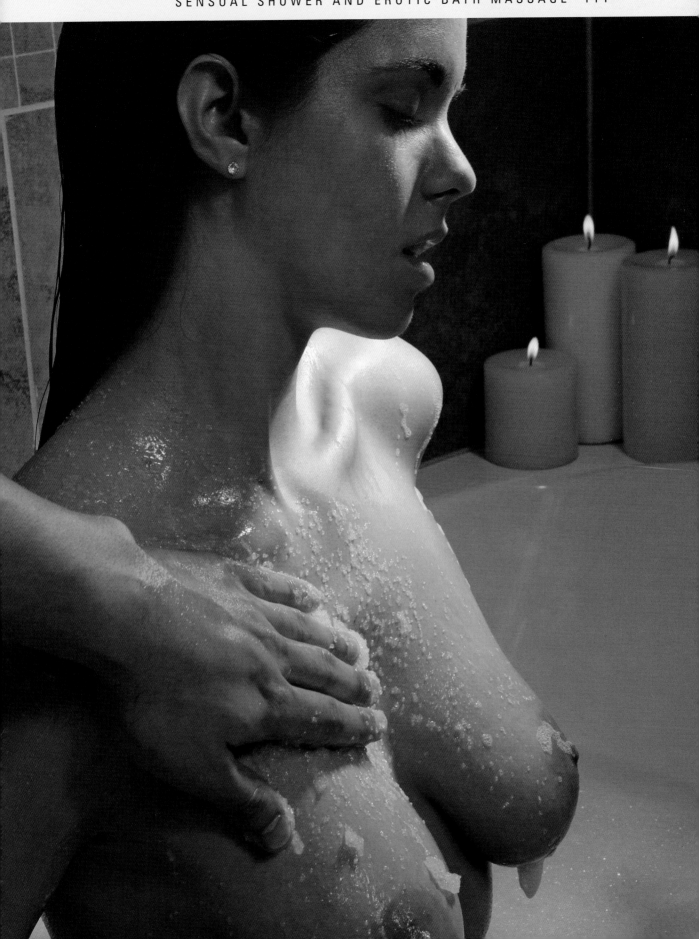

Anoint Her with Scented Oils

Scented oils are an additional way to enhance the smell and feel of the skin. I recommend ylang-ylang, sandalwood, lavender, rose, and citrus oils. These exotic scents help awaken the sexual centers. Place a little oil on your fingertip, and touch her under her nose to leave a trace. When massaging her breast, stimulate her olfactory sense with rose oil. You may wish to anoint each breast with rose oil—the oil of nurturance and love.

When you get to the head, have her inhale lavender oil, and anoint her middle forehead with this precious oil of peace and serenity. Anoint as if you were a king, and perhaps give her a spontaneous blessing. Our sense of smell is the most primitive of our senses, and it awakens deep memories and passions.

Bless Her Breasts and Genitals

Wash the scented oils from your hands and ask for permission to touch her intimate parts. Slip a bar of soap over her curves and between her legs. Lift her pelvis partway out of the water, if possible, for more play. Keep soap and scented oils out of the vagina and save internal massage for later. Slip your fingers down the inner lips and massage the perineum with a couple of flat fingers. Circle the clitoris and vaginal opening with light and teasing fingers and slippery soap.

Melted Love in Your Hands

Bathe your partner's back and neck by sitting her up and bending her forward slightly. End with a gentle face caress and a head massage. After bathing her for about forty minutes, gently help her step out of the tub. Dry her off with a towel and dress her in a robe. Escort her to the room in which you will continue her full body massage. A long, hot bath turns your lover into a baby; she's putty in your arms for the massage.

Letting one stroke lead into another in a continuous fluid dance, massage her back side, then front side, then ask for permission to honor her genitals. Twenty to thirty minutes works well for each segment. After you've completed the massage, continue erotic play if both of you desire, sip wine, plan time to spoon together, or just fall asleep.

Heaven for Him

For a man, receiving a perineum massage in a hot bath is heaven. Pull up on the scrotum and with a fist, press into the perineum. Men often think they need to be hard if a woman is touching them, but women relate to a man's vulnerability and enjoy his many stages of arousal. A woman connects with a man when he can relax about being soft, medium-hard, or hard. When he lets go of pressuring himself, he can enjoy subtle arousal ripples. Accept the situation and be present in the moment.

RUB-A-DUB-DUB, TWO IN THE TUB

A fun variation is to take turns bathing each other while sharing a bath. This mutual play changes the character of the bath ritual. The bath becomes less nurturing for the receiver and more playful and erotic.

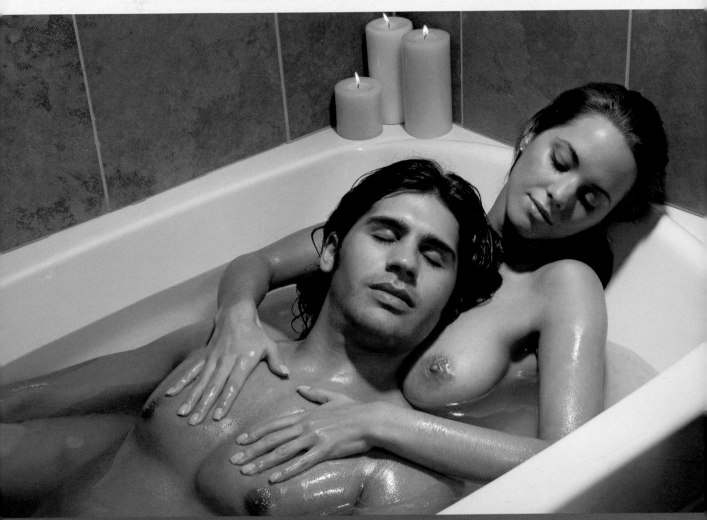

A long, hot bath turns your lover into a baby;
he'll be putty in your arms for the massage.

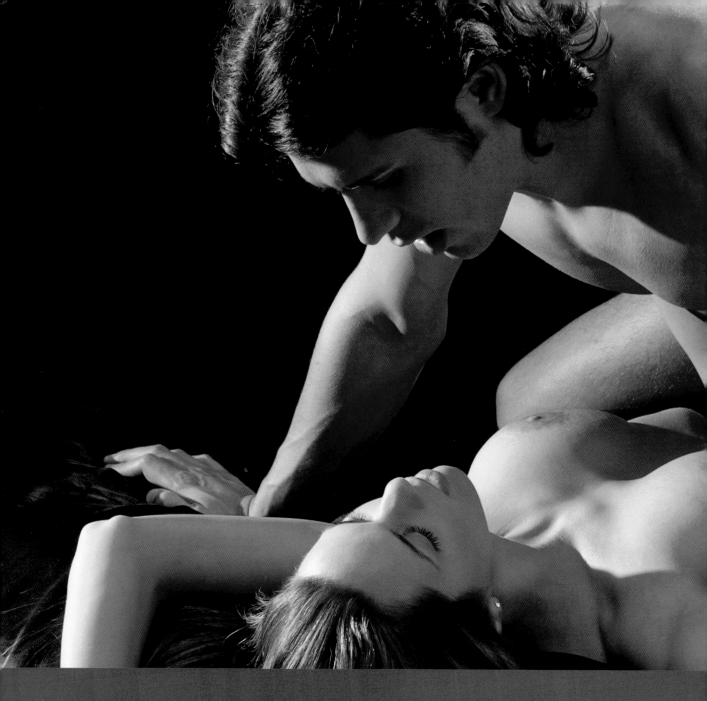

chapter
EIGHT

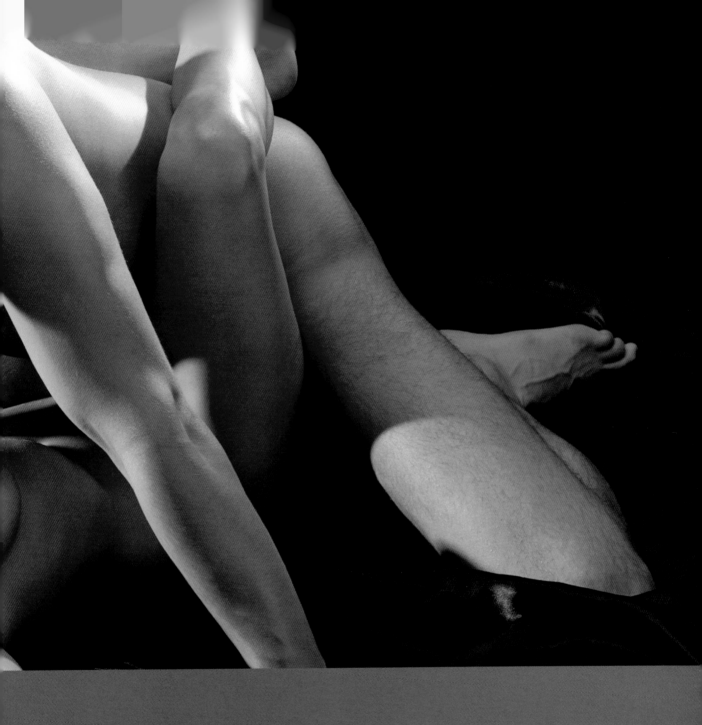

KISSING, ORAL SEX, AND INTERCOURSE

TENDER KISSES

One of the surest ways you can tell if you want to go further with a partner is to test the waters with kissing. If a man or a woman is too eager, and rushes past the subtle and whispery beginnings, you need to slow the pace. Immediate hard and wet mouth mauling misses the point. Discovery by tongue is a tender, playful journey.

Start out slowly and leisurely with your kissing. How lightly can you kiss? With a relaxed, soft mouth, graze over his cheeks and facial features by barely touching the skin. Trace the eyebrows with soft lips. Tenderly kiss the tip of his nose and the corners of his lips. The mouth, not your hand, becomes the sensate-focus tool.

Breathe lightly into an ear and lick its contour. The mouth is so sensitive that less is often more. Your lips and tongue are exploring and discovering each nook and mound. Your attitude is inquisitive—playing a new game with each kiss. Once you reach his mouth, kiss lightly without your tongue at first.

THE KISSING GAME

At one time in my life, I had the most wonderful kisser for a boyfriend, so I was surprised when after time I got bored with our kissing. Then I discovered why. He was always kissing me (active) and I was always receiving his gestures. As soon as I realized I needed to be more active in this game, things cooked up. Instead of the predictable "his way," we began to share the lead. Culturally, women are shy to lead, but men love it. They really want to please us and are thankful when we show them how.

Here's a nonverbal kissing game to try with your partner. Take turns being the active kisser and the receiver of kisses, or "kissee." When you are the kissee, offer a soft, slightly open mouth for the kisser's exploration and do not react by moving. Close your eyes and tune in to your sensations. Breathe. When you are the kisser, find new ways to explore the sensations of your mouth and tongue for your pleasure on your lover's face and body. Tune in to your sensations and breathe. Decide on a time frame, such as ten minutes, then switch roles. Afterward, talk about what you liked most about your partner's kisses.

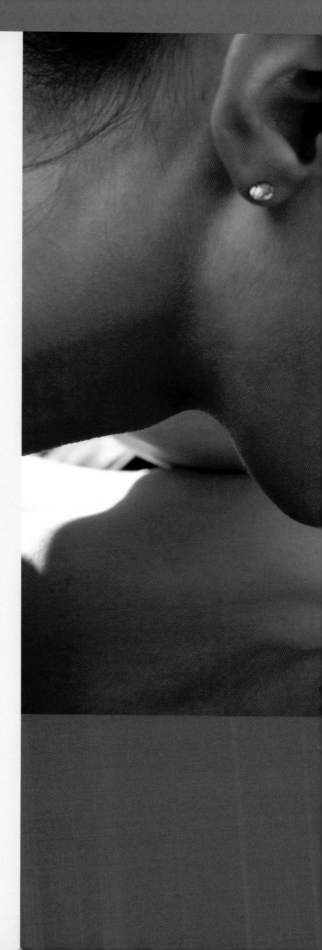

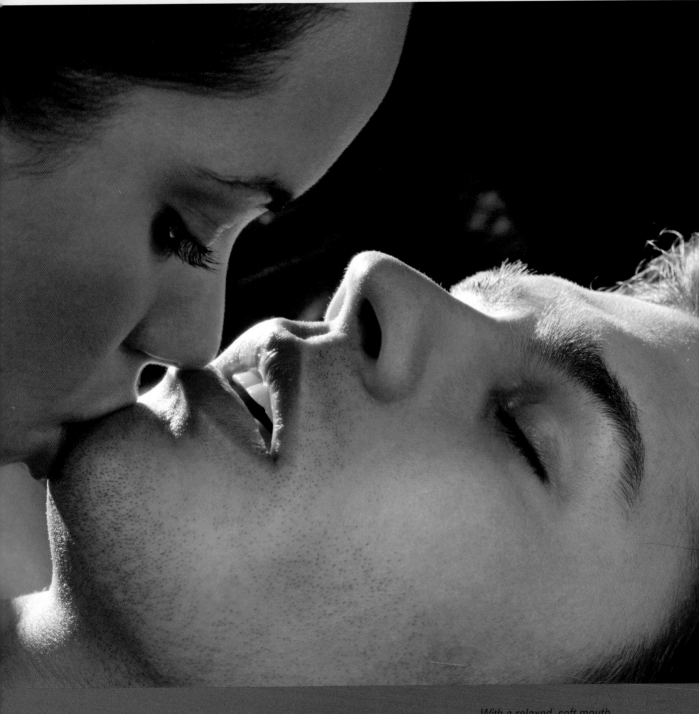

With a relaxed, soft mouth, delicately graze your lips over his cheeks and face.

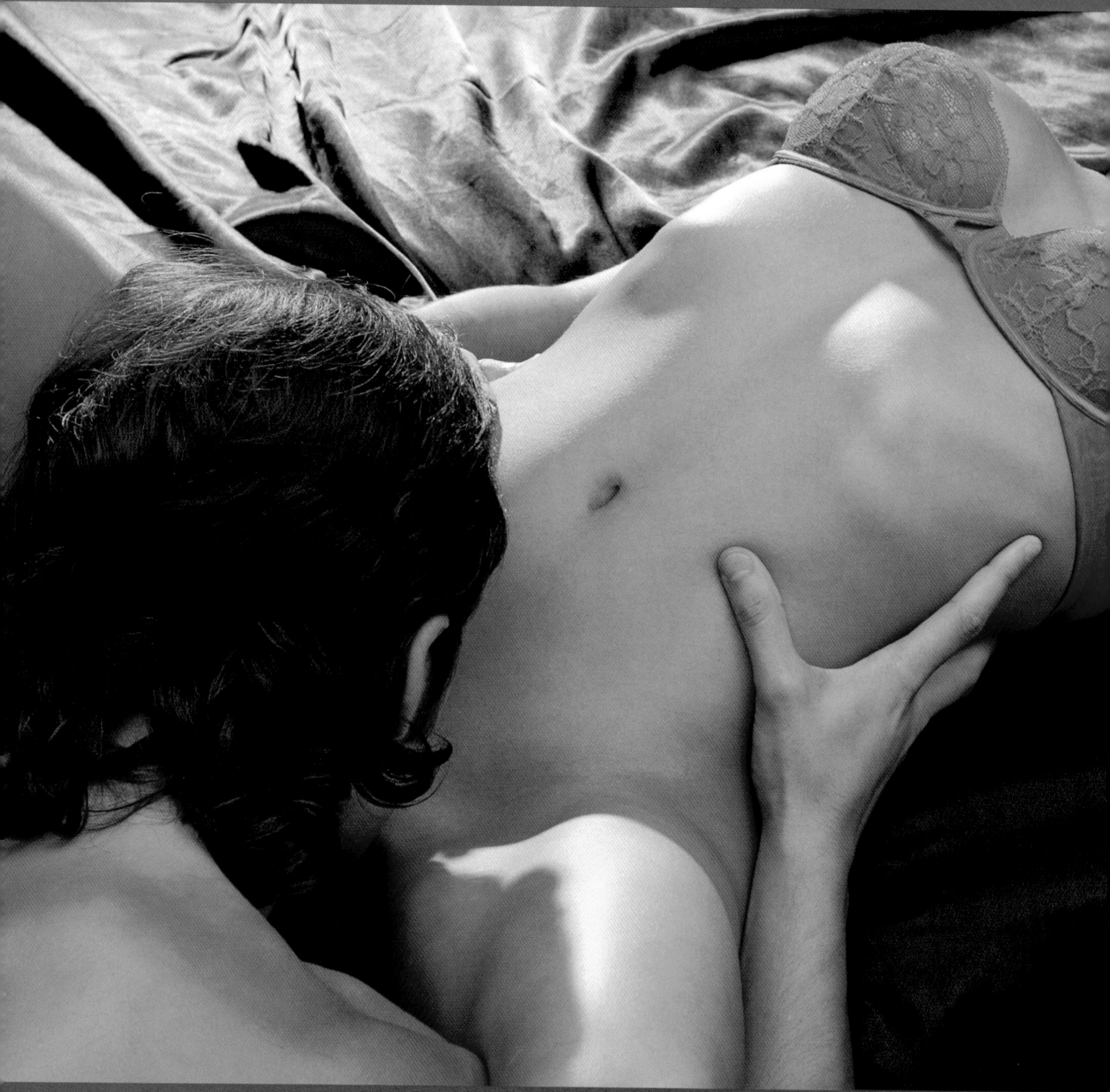

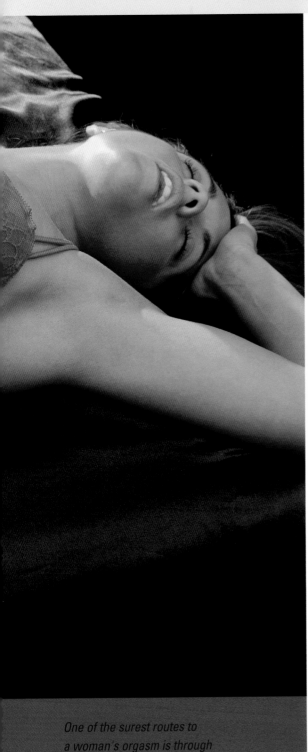

One of the surest routes to a woman's orgasm is through oral sex.

SPECIAL KISSES

For variety, try some *fruity kisses*. Blindfold your partner and have slices of fresh fruit to share with him when you are the active one in the kissing game. Rub his lips with pineapple, running the cool, textured sweetness over his lips. Lick the juice off his lips. Tease a raspberry onto his tongue. Loll it gently around with your tongue. Bite into a slice of mango and feather it into his mouth. Share in the juices. Switch roles.

Another oral delight is *body tasting*, where you apply your favorite food to your lover's body only to be licked off by you. Whipped cream, honey, and chocolate sauce are some favorites. Savor the flavors mixed with your lover's essence. Take turns and take your time. Do not place any food in the vagina, and leave time for a sensual shower afterward. Perhaps an old sheet and kitchen table would be ideal for your feast.

ORAL SEX

An unfortunate myth of our time is that a penis-in-the vagina sex is sufficient stimulation to bring a woman to orgasm. However, rarely is intercourse alone enough stimulation of the clitoris to bring a woman to climax. When a man becomes skillful at oral pleasuring techniques, he becomes her hero.

CUNNILINGUS

Make sure you are in a comfortable position for cunnilingus, and project to your woman the honest feeling that you want to be there—for as long as she will allow you. If you lick and suck her for the pleasure it brings you, she will sense it and allow you to play down there. If she feels you are trying to make her come, she'll feel pressured and worry that she is too slow, which suppresses her orgasm. If you stay with what gives you real delight, she is free to feel her own enjoyment. Don't make orgasm your goal. Remember, orgasm is something we allow ourselves, it is not something we "give" to another person. So relax, enjoy the ride, and she will, too.

Play with a delicate, soft, wet tongue, varying the rhythm and the pressure. Lap the area with a flat, broad tongue. Circle the clitoris with a wet tongue, enclose it with your mouth , and suck on it with little kisses. Once you've lubricated the clitoris, slide your tongue slowly down to the opening of the vagina and, using an erect tongue, probe the opening.

Pleasure Blocks

Be aware of blocks that hinder some women from enjoying oral sex. She may fear that her genitals are ugly, or that they don't smell good, or that it will take her too long to orgasm. Be sure to compliment your woman on how beautiful you find her vagina, describing its beauty as an orchid flower, for example. Genital juices for both men and women are an acquired taste. Take a shower together before oral sex if her unique scent isn't pleasing to you. After a few tongue explorations, tell her how sweet she tastes.

Sexual Bonding

While spooning with your partner, insert a soft or hard penis into the vagina and stay connected in stillness without moving for twenty minutes. Feel the sexual ripples appear and disappear. Tune in to the breath, whole-body peace, and the subtle joy of no pressure to perform. You might even try falling asleep connected.

Ascent to Orgasm

When the vagina is relaxed and silky, slide one or two fingers inside. Hold still at first, as the energy from penetration is intense, then move your finger(s) slowly back and forth. Keep playing with her clitoris with your mouth. To give your jaw a rest, you can alternate between oral sex and using your hand in the vagina. Move your hand slowly and press your finger(s) toward the ceiling of her vagina. Gently rub the G-spot in a come-hither gesture, while still paying frequent oral attention to the clitoris.

On her ascent to orgasm, don't become overzealous. Her sighs most likely signal that what you're doing is just right, not that she needs more. Maintain your consistency and steadiness without speeding up or changing stimulation, which can throw her off. After orgasm, both men and women become hypersensitive, so lighten the touch, staying with her and discerning whether or not she would like to go for another orgasm.

FELLATIO

When a man shows up for a woman, caresses her with his attention, and consciously connects with her from his heart space, she wants to take more of him inside her. When a man adores a woman, touches her unhurriedly, has good oral and manual skills, uses lube on her clitoris, and can ask how she likes to be touched, she adores him. A man who knows the value of slow penetration (with eyes, fingers, or penis), can talk about sex, and explores ways to make it better, can cuddle in the afterglow of closeness, is rewarded by a turned-on woman who wants to go down on him.

There is no one right way to orally pleasure your man. Do what pleases you for as long as it pleases you, then find something else to do. You don't have to swallow ejaculate or even bring him to climax. You suck his penis because it feels good to your tongue and the sucking motion makes you also feel juicy, sexy, and turned on. No contract to fulfill here, no prescribed outcome, just play. You're in charge.

Enjoy the different sensations of the shaft and the head of the penis, and include his scrotum and nipples if you like. To give your mouth a rest, alternate between mouth and hand stimulation. Try combining hand and mouth massage for a different sensation. With one hand holding the base of the penis, pull the skin taut at the head, which increases sensation, then play with the head in your mouth. Tell him how good he tastes and how beautiful he is.

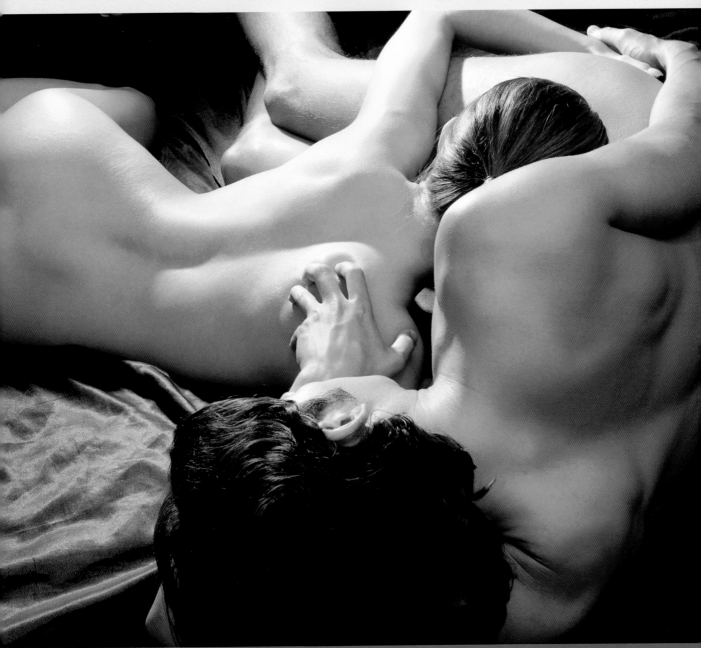

"*When I finally started going down on my boyfriend with my pleasure in mind, something snapped. I became free and loved it. Now I design the show for me and he loves it. Each time is different because my expectations are gone.*"
—*Claire, 27*

When men show up for women and connect with them from the heart, women offer them a world of pleasure.

INTERCOURSE:
ANOTHER WAY TO TOUCH

Intercourse is simply another form of touching. Because we have elevated it to the ultimate experience, and rush down a direct path to its door, we often forget to relish the experiences along the way. The caresses and massages in this book are the sensual experiences that make intercourse desirable, and I hope they have already changed your approach to it.

The play so prevalent and exciting to us as teenagers often vanishes for us when we become adults. Sexuality was magical in our adolescent years when we wandered aimlessly into pleasure, but as adults it became serious and focused.

Generally, men tend to direct sex play with goal-oriented results in mind—intercourse and ejaculation. Women, naturally indirect and meandering in their approach, have not committed to initiating and directing sexual encounters to fit their needs. *When women commit to co-create as equal consorts in the game of lovemaking, everything changes.*

This book is about trusting the dance between equals. By taking turns giving and receiving, we harmonize the male and the female within each of us. Unless you have skipped directly to this chapter, the book's exercises have probably transformed the way you make love. By including the whole body in touch, touching with more skill and less expectation, practicing deep breathing and presence, you restore balance and authenticity in your sex life.

THE WOMAN ACTIVE

After you have massaged and caressed for some time, lay him on his back and straddle his pelvis with your hips. The woman on top gives you control of the timing, rhythm, depth and range of motion. He is "being done" and will not "take over." Although men often feel they need to be in the driver's seat after a while, remind him to lie back and enjoy the ride.

When you feel ready, lubricate his penis (flaccid or hard) and massage your vulva with it. Gaze into each other's eyes and connect in the breath. Guide his penis into your lips and vagina, holding him in with your PC muscle or nestling him between your vaginal lips. With your other hand, stroke his chest, shoulders, hips, and thighs. Move however the spirit moves you. Lift up, circle, and gyrate your hips in a slow, undulating dance. There is no right way to do intercourse. He doesn't need to be hard, and intercourse doesn't have to end in orgasm. If you want to stimulate your clitoris with your own hand, do it. If you want to use a vibrator between you and your partner, do it. Orgasming together is no more right than orgasming at different times, or not at all. Ending intercourse without orgasm doesn't mean you have a low libido, it means you are present and respectful of your desires.

Orgasm is a personal experience in a sea of togetherness. While the ascent to orgasm is supported by your partner, it is essentially an individual experience. It is natural to feel separate or self-absorbed at the moment of climax.

Saying Yes and Saying No for Women

Intercourse as obligation, a bargaining chip, or even to save a relationship, creates distance and numbs the body. Being true to your desires, on the other hand, is invigorating. Pleasure, not pretending, is what's important. Being able to say no is an integral part of building trust and intimacy in a relationship.

Conversely, sometimes women have a hard time saying yes when they want something (or taking the lead in sex). Women are often afraid of seeming too wanton, sluttish, or morally loose. However, a big turnon for a man is being with a turned-on woman. Nothing is hotter than a woman taking control of her pleasure. Being able to clearly say no and yes is a gift to yourself, your partner, and your passions.

THE MAN ACTIVE

After a quality whole body massage, leisurely stroke the woman's entire vulva using massage oil. Don't focus on the clitoris yet. You're letting desire build slowly, not trying to get her hot. Shift to oral sex by rolling your tongue over the clitoris and moistening the vaginal opening.

After at least five minutes on the clitoris, press the pad of your finger over the vagina to check for wetness; if she feels dry, add lubrication. Be a tease, step up, step back. The most sensitive part of the vagina is the opening; spend time there, circling it with your fingers. Slowly ease one finger into the vagina, bit by bit. Do you feel suction or friction? Play around till you feel her "pulling you in." Add a second finger to prepare her for the girth of your penis.

Position yourself to penetrate her vagina while you continue to manually stimulate her clitoris. While nudging the head of your penis ever so slightly against the dip at the opening of her vagina, ask her to squeeze and release her PC muscle, which helps relax the vaginal muscles. Move inside little by little. Rarely are women penetrated slowly and sensuously enough to create deep pleasure. The mushroom head of your penis is perfect for massaging the G-spot through slow, seamless, shallow penetration.

Be aware of your conditioning to think it is your responsibility to give her an orgasm. If your self-esteem hinges on her orgasm, she will feel the pressure. Better to encourage her to enjoy each moment for its own wonder.

"My husband and I were in a sexual rut——no foreplay and straight to sex, and not lasting very long at it before he climaxed. I decided to take matters into my own hands. I began to flirt with him, get him hot with my words, and play with him sexually to my heart's desire——always stopping short of letting him come. I felt his attention and desire for me build and mine for him, too. These teasing turnon sessions without intercourse (by my design!) made for explosive sex when we were both ready. The randomness of intercourse increased the quality of his attention to me. I began receiving flowers and jewelry. A new interest and sweetness marked our marriage."

—Veronica, 37

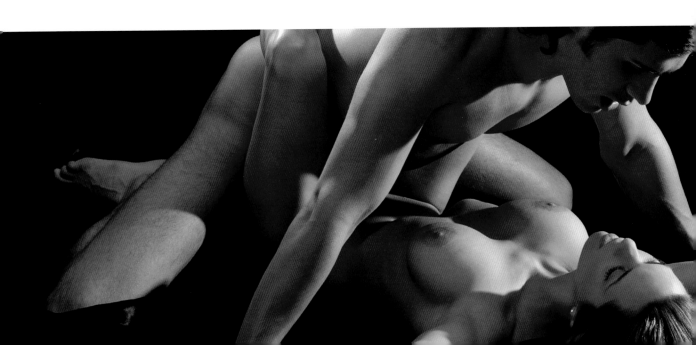

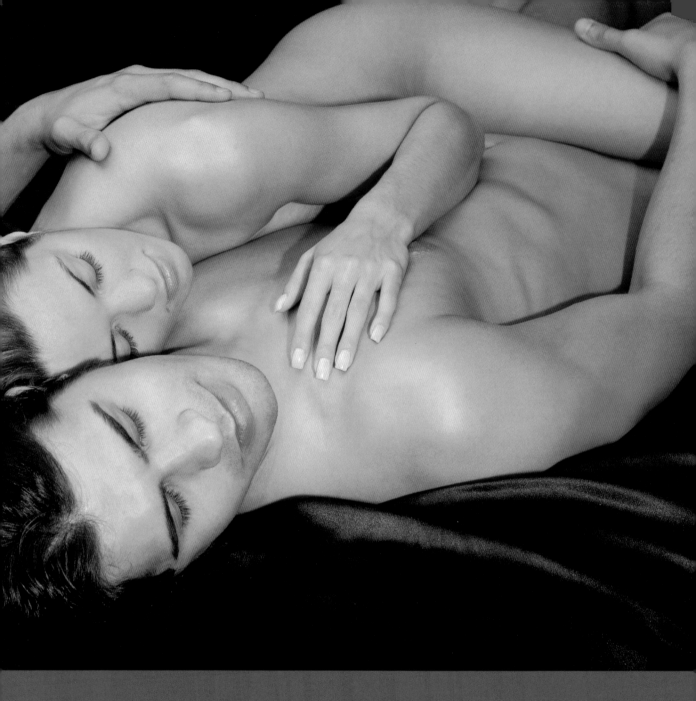

chapter

NINE